TRADI

Chinese Medicine

Richard Craze

with

Jen T'ieh Fou

TEACH YOURSELF BOOKS

This book is dedicated to Sally Craze.

And with very grateful thanks to Jen T'ieh Fou, Consultant editor, for checking the technical information in this book.

The author would also like to thank all the Chinese doctors who have gone before and charted this fascinating subject.

Jen T'ieh Fou is an acupuncturist and teacher of Chinese medicine practising in the UK.

Long-renowned as the authoritative source for self-guided learning – with more than 30 million copies sold worldwide – the *Teach Yourself* series includes over 200 titles in the fields of languages, crafts, hobbies, sports, and other leisure activities.

A catalogue record for this title is available from the British Library.

Library of Congress Catalog Card Number: on file.

First published in UK 1998 by Hodder Headline Plc, 338 Euston Road, London NW1 3BH

First published in US 1998 by NTC Publishing Group
An imprint of NTC/Contemporary Publishing Company
4255 West Touhy Avenue, Lincolnwood (Chicago), Illinois 60646-1975 U.S.A.

The 'Teach Yourself' name and logo are registered trade marks of Hodder & Stoughton Ltd in the UK.

Typeset by Transet Limited, Coventry, England.
Printed in England by Cox & Wyman Limited, Reading, Berkshire.

Impression number   10 9 8 7 6 5 4 3 2 1
Year   2002 2001 2000 1999 1998

CONTENTS

INTRODUCTION

The Tao that can be trodden is not the enduring and unchanging Tao. The name that can be named is not the enduring and unchanging name.

Tao Ti Ching

When I first said I was writing a book entitled *Teach Yourself Traditional Chinese Medicine* there were lots of jokes about people practising acupuncture on themselves at home. So let's clear up a couple of things before we go any further. This is not a book about how to practise any forms of Chinese medicine on yourself. Nor is it intended as any sort of diagnostic manual. So who is it for? And what is it for?

This book is intended for several different categories of people:

- Anyone who would like to learn how to stay fit and healthy according to Chinese principles
- Anyone with a general interest in Chinese culture and tradition
- Anyone embarking on a course of Chinese medicine who would like to know what they are going to experience and what sort of results they can expect
- Anyone studying Chinese medicine either with the intention of becoming a practitioner themselves or for research purposes
- Teachers of Chinese medicine
- Professionals working within Western medicine who wish to expand their knowledge of Chinese medicine
- Anyone with a friend or relative who is undergoing a course of Chinese medicine.

This is, however, not a book of do-it-yourself diagnostics, remedies or treatment. Yes, you may well be able to find your particular disorder listed and described but this book is not intended to take the place of a qualified practitioner of Chinese medicine. It has to be said that if you are in any doubt as to your health or medical history then you should consult a doctor immediately.

This book is intended to be accessible to the lay person so the technical information has been made as simple as possible while retaining its comprehensiveness. However, Chapters 5 and 7 have been written more with students of Chinese medicine in mind. The Appendices, too, will probably be of more interest to students and practitioners than to the beginner.

So what is traditional Chinese medicine? Here in the West we are likely to think of it as being merely acupuncture and that's something to do with sticking pins in people, isn't it? Well, no. There is a vast range of disciplines within Chinese medicine which include:

- Herbal medicine
- Acupuncture
- Acupressure
- Moxibustion
- Massage
- Preventative medicine
- Medicinal foods
- Ch'i Kung
- Tui Na
- Tai Ch'i.

Chinese medicine has been practised for at least five centuries, making it one of the oldest medical disciplines in the world. Some of the earliest medical textbooks are Chinese, including the Yellow Emperor's Classic of Internal Medicine (the *Huang-ti Nei Ching Su Wen*), which was written in the third century BC. This is probably the world's oldest textbook, and it is also still in print and in current usage.

In 1973 a 2,100-year-old tomb in China's Hunan Province was opened and found to contain a set of medical textbooks printed on silk that outlined the principles of Chinese medicine including pulse-taking, yin and yang and diagnostic techniques.

It is known that acupuncture was practised in the Stone Age using slivers of stone and bone called *bian*. By the eighth century BC metal needles were being used, and by around 3000 BC gold needles had been introduced. Remains of these have been excavated from tombs in the Hubei Province: gold acupuncture needles over 5,000 years old.

So why isn't more known about these medical techniques in the West? Well, for many centuries China kept herself very isolated from the rest of the world. A small inroad was made by the Jesuit priests from around 1850 but the barriers came down again during the Cultural Revolution and it has only been in the last 30 years that the West has had access to the vast storehouses of information that make up Chinese medicine.

Basic principles

Chinese medicine is quite unlike Western medicine in that it deals with a different concept of the human body. Western medicine doesn't recognise some of the fundamental principles behind Chinese medicine such as meridians, ch'i energy, the five elements and the concept of yin and yang. That situation, however, is rapidly changing.

The meridians

Chinese medical practitioners hold that energy flows through the body along 12 energy paths known as meridians. These are not the conventional blood vessels, nor are they nerves, but a total different set of pathways. The energy that flows along the meridians is ch'i and it is capable of being blocked, stagnating, being weakened and having its flow reversed. All these conditions will result in the ill health of the patient. By manipulating the meridians at certain energy crossovers or meridian points, the acupuncturist can restore the flow of energy and thus also the health of the patient.

Ch'i energy

Ch'i is the universal energy. It flows within, around and through all things in the universe, including us. When the flow is not harmonious it causes us ill health. The art of manipulating the flow of ch'i energy externally through and within our living space is known as Feng Shui (wind and water). Ch'i cannot be destroyed but it can be negatively affected. Each organ in the human body has its own type of ch'i, as does blood, body fluids, breath and digestion. By keeping a close eye on the flow of ch'i within the human body the Chinese medical practitioner can help maintain health. They monitor the flow of ch'i by regularly taking the patient's pulses. In the West we are used to the notion of a single pulse being taken in either wrist, but a Chinese practitioner will take up to six pulses in each wrist.

The five elements

According to traditional Chinese philosophy everything in the universe can be broken down into one of five basic parts – the five elements, which are water, fire, earth, metal and wood. When there is an imbalance of any of these within the human body there is a resulting loss of good health. By restoring the balance, usually by prescribing herbal remedies, the practitioner can also restore the health of the patient.

Yin and yang

These are the two fundamental principles or concepts behind which the whole of Chinese philosophy is based. The two are not opposing forces as in right and wrong, but are complementary – without one you cannot have the other. They are often seen as male and female or positive and negative. But that is to limit them too much. They are the complementary forces in everything – day and night, heat and cold, dry and wet, winter and summer, life and death, rising and falling, declining and growing. When there is an imbalance of one or the other the patient can experience ill health and the Chinese medical practitioner will work hard to restore the balance.

The main forms of Chinese medicine

Chinese medical practitioners don't tend to be quite so specialist in their outlook as their Western counterparts. They tend to use whatever technique is available to help the patient and as they all agree on the fundamental principles behind medicine they can switch easily from one discipline to another. The main forms of Chinese medicine are:

- herbalism
- acupuncture
- moxibustion
- acupressure
- Ch'i Kung
- massage

Herbalism

This is the use of herbs to balance the yin and yang and to improve or restore the flow of ch'i. The herbs are usually taken internally (although some are applied as skin ointments) and in combinations of up to 12 individual herbs. Nearly all of the herbs used are grown, prepared and packaged in mainland China or Hong Kong. They are not particularly similar to Western herbs as most of them are used in a dried or prepared state whereas most Western herbs are used fresh. Chinese herbs are more similar to Western generic medicines, some even coming in the form of pills, ointments or liquid medicines.

Chinese herbal medicines are usually given in combinations. These combinations are based on a variety of factors:

- *Complements.* Two or more herbs of similar properties and effects are used together to increase their desired beneficial quality.
- *Assistants.* Two or more herbs of different properties and effects are used in combination. One herb has the main medicinal effect required while the other has a catalytic function to increase the effectiveness of the first.
- *Frights.* One herb is used to moderate the action of another to lessen any dangerous side-effects.
- *Hates.* One herb is used to modify another's effects so as to achieve the desired result.
- *Cancellations.* If a herb has inconvenient, though not dangerous, side-effects, a second herb may be used to cancel these out.
- *Contrasts.* This is a deliberate mis-combination of two herbs that result in violent bodily reactions, rarely prescribed.

Chinese oral herbal medicines are generally prescribed to be drunk as a soup or a tea.

Acupuncture

The ch'i energy flows along the 12 meridians to all parts of the body to produce harmonious health and growth. Sometimes the meridians, for various reasons including emotional trauma, infections, poor diet, injury or illness, become blocked and the ch'i flow becomes restricted. The whole body can then go into a decline and the original blockage can be difficult to locate. By using metal needles inserted into the meridian lines at specific acupoints the acupuncturist clears the blockage and restores the flow of ch'i, thus restoring the health of the individual. Over 2,000 acupoints have been established but most acupuncturists use on average around 150 (although most treatments wouldn't use more than two or three in any one session).

Moxibustion

Sometimes when the acupuncturist wants to supplement or tone the energy they will use the technique known as moxibustion. This is when a glowing ember of the herb *Artemesia japonica* (*also known as Artemesia vulgaris latiflora*) is used to apply gentle heat to an acupoint. The herb may be burnt in small cones on the skin directly or on the handle of an acupuncture needle to transfer the heat directly into the meridian. The glowing ember is removed when the patient can feel the heat, so there is no question of a burn resulting.

Acupressure

If the patient has an aversion to needles, or a fear of the pain that they think they may suffer, or an allergy or blood disorder that would prevent the insertion of needles, then the acupuncturist will apply a gentle pressure using their fingers to the acupoint instead of a needle. This is called acupressure and seems to have the same effect as inserting a needle, except that it is slower-acting, less direct and less guaranteed in results. It is a treatment especially suitable for children.

Ch'i Kung

Ch'i Kung (sometimes spelt *qi gong*) is used in China as a method of preventing illness and promoting good health. It is based on a series of physical and meditative exercises that help the flow of ch'i. It involves some breathing exercises, some martial arts type movements (it is sometimes used as a martial art in China) and some relaxation exercises. It is suitable for all age groups and is thought to be especially beneficial to people recovering from illness as it strengthens ch'i and quickly restores health. It is usually practised for about 15 minutes once a day.

Massage

Chinese medicine practitioners will sometimes decide that the whole body of the patient needs to be massaged to restore the flow of ch'i.

Sometimes they will only massage specific points like the shoulders or the back of the neck. It is almost like acupressure: moving the ch'i along the meridians by stimulating the skin and muscles. It is very similar to Shiatsu, the Japanese massage technique. It is often referred to as Shen Dao or Ch'i Shu or Tui Na.

In *Teach Yourself Traditional Chinese Medicine* we will look at both the theory and practice – how it is done and why it is done. And we shall also look at the most common disorders and diseases that Chinese medicine is likely to treat. These range from simple disorders like the common cold to complex conditions such as infertility and alcoholism. Always remember, though, that this is not a book of self-diagnosis and the conditions with their respective treatments are there for information only. If you suspect that you are suffering from any particular condition you must seek medical advice immediately. This is a reference book not a book designed to take the place of your doctor. When using any treatments at home please exercise extreme caution. For instance Chinese herbal medicine uses some very potent remedies which if taken in excess would be extremely dangerous as they are very concentrated. Under no circumstances should any course of treatment be taken on the grounds that it was prescribed for someone else with a similar ailment.

The difference between Western and Eastern medicine

Chinese medicine is very different from any branch of Western medicine; the fundamental differences of philosophy, diagnosis and approach are vast. This book sets out to explain to Western readers exactly what those differences are and how traditional Chinese medicine works. There are three main differences between Chinese medicine and conventional Western treatments that will be explored. They can be seen simply as:

- Chinese medicine treats the whole person rather than just the complaint;
- Chinese medicine regards herbs, correctly used, as benign rather than as potions or poisons;
- Chinese medicine is primarily a preventative rather than curative discipline.

── The World Health Organisation ──

The World Health Organisation (WHO) has published a list of ailments for which Chinese medicine is considered appropriate treatment. They include:

- infections – colds and flu, bronchitis, hepatitis;
- internal – hypoglycaemia, asthma, high blood pressure, ulcers, colitis, indigestion, haemorrhoids, diarrhoea, constipation, diabetes;
- eyes, ears, nose and throat – deafness, ringing in the ears, earaches, poor eyesight, dizziness, sinus infection, sore throat, hay fever;
- dermatological – eczema, acne, herpes;
- muscular, skeletal and neurologic – arthritis, neuralgia, sciatica, back pain, bursitis, tendonitis, stiff neck, Bell's palsy, trigeminal neuralgia, headache, stroke, cerebral palsy, polio, sprains;
- mental-emotional – anxiety, depression, stress, insomnia;
- genito-urinary and reproductive – impotence, infertility, pre-menstrual syndrome (PMS), pelvic inflammatory disease (PID), vaginitis, irregular period or cramps, morning sickness.

A World Health Organisation interregional seminar on acupuncture, moxibustion and acupuncture anaesthesia was held in Beijing in June 1979, attended by participants from 12 countries. Its purpose was to discuss ways in which priorities and standards could be determined in the acupuncture areas of clinical work, research, training, and technology transfer. Scientific investigation must be closely correlated with demonstrations of acupuncture's clinical efficacy. Apart from acupuncture analgesia used in major surgical procedures, acupuncture also has been applied as a diagnostic aid and in conjunction with fluoroscopy in gastro-intestinal diseases. Acupuncture is clearly not a panacea; but the sheer weight of evidence demands that acupuncture must be taken seriously as a clinical procedure of considerable value.

During the past decade, there has been a growing convergence between the most advanced research knowledge from physiology, biochemistry and pharmacology, and knowledge obtained by research in the field of acupuncture; that is to say, a convergence of modern international science with traditional Chinese medicine. For example, in more than 600 cases of coronary heart disease, the effectiveness of acupuncture in relieving the symptoms was over 80 per cent. In 645 cases of acute bacillary dysentery, 90 per cent of the patients were cured within ten days as judged by clinical symptoms and signs and the results of stool culture. The technique is also comparatively effective in controlling fever, inflammation and pain.

From the viewpoint of modern medicine, the principle action of acupuncture (and of moxibustion) is to regulate the function of the human body and to increase its resistance by enhancing the immune system and the antiphlogistic, analgesic, antispastic, antishock and antiparalytic abilities of the body.

The World Health Organisation Interregional Seminar drew up the following provisional list of diseases that lend themselves to acupuncture treatment. The list is based on clinical experience, and not necessarily on controlled clinical research: furthermore, the inclusion of specific diseases are not meant to indicate the extent of acupuncture's efficacy in treating them.

Upper respiratory tract

Acute sinusitis
Acute rhinitis
Common cold
Acute tonsillitis

Respiratory system

Acute bronchitis
Bronchial asthma (most effective in children and in patients without complicating diseases)

Eye disorders

Acute conjunctivitis
Central retinitis
Myopia (in children)
Cataract (without complications)

Disorders of the mouth

Toothache, post-extraction pain
Gingivitis
Acute and chronic pharyngitis

Gastro-intestinal disorders

Spasms of oesophagus and cardia
Hiccoughs
Gastroptosis
Acute and chronic gastritis
Gastric hyperacidity
Chronic duodenal ulcer (pain relief)
Acute duodenal ulcer (without complications)
Acute and chronic colitis
Acute bacillary dysentery
Constipation
Diarrhoea
Paralytic ileus

Neurological and musculo-skeletal disorders

Headache and migraine
Trigeminal neuralgia
Facial palsy (early stage, i.e. within 3–6 months)
Pareses following a stroke
Peripheral neuropathies
Sequelae of poliomyelitis (early stage, i.e. within 6 months)
Meniere's disease
Neurogenic bladder dysfunction
Nocturnal enuresis (bed-wetting)
Intercostal neuralgia
Cervicobrachial syndrome
'Frozen shoulder,' 'tennis elbow'
Sciatica
Low back pain
Osteoarthritis

—— Growing interest in the West ——

Chinese medicine provides primary health care for a quarter to a half of the world's population. It is practised in more than a dozen National Health Service clinics in the UK already.

The growing interest in the West is not based on a whim but on results. Ten years ago in the UK there were only a handful of Chinese medical practitioners. Now there are over five hundred. They rarely advertise, relying on word of mouth for most of their business. That business is growing each year because of the results obtained.

In the US over $400 million is spent each year on Chinese medicine, while in Germany the figure is estimated at $1.5 billion.

——— The Chinese practitioner ———

A Chinese medical practitioner may also be qualified for acupuncture, herbalism or any of the other forms of Chinese medicine. They may have trained in China or in the West and should hold an officially recognised qualification and belong to a professional register.

A consultation with a practitioner will usually begin with a full investigation of the patient's past medical history and an examination using the four traditional diagnostic techniques:

- *Looking.* Observing the patient's facial colour, general body type and language, the appearance of the tongue, mental state and expression.
- *Feeling.* The Chinese practitioner feels for three pulses in each wrist which indicate the functioning of the major organs and for the palpation of the flow of ch'i (energy).
- *Listening.* Listening to the patient's breathing, coughing and voice.
- *Asking.* Finding out the patient's full medical history, their lifestyle, their diet, sex life, fears and upbringing.

CAUTION

In the hands of an experienced, qualified practitioner traditional Chinese medicine can sometimes be used to treat serious, even life-threatening illnesses. It should never be used in that way by anyone else.

Self-diagnosis and treatment should only be used for the most minor of ailments, and a doctor should be consulted immediately if any symptoms persist or become aggravated. Any other symptoms such as high or low temperature, delirium or any other indication that the illness is anything more than a minor complaint should be reported to a doctor immediately.

Many of the herbs contained in the book refer to the wild native Chinese variety which are obtainable from reputable herbal

---

stockists. They are not to be confused with any Western herbs that sound, look or taste similar. Even using another species of the same herbal family will not produce the same results and may even be positively dangerous.

Chinese spelling

Originally in the West we have used a system of Chinese spelling which gave us such examples as Peking. Now the system has changed and the new system – called *pin-yin* – gives us Beijing instead. It also changes *ch'i* to *qi*. I have used mostly the Wade Giles system as the pin-yin seems unfamiliar and somehow awkward. I have, however, used the pin-yin for major place names such as Beijing.

1

THE PHILOSOPHY OF CHINESE MEDICINE

Always without desire we must be found,
If its deep mystery we would sound;
But if desire always within us be,
Its outer fringe is all that we shall see.

Tao Ti Ching

To understand the principles of Chinese medicine we have to have an understanding of Taoism, the religion of China. Taoism comes from the Tao (pronounced *Dow*), meaning the Way. The Chinese say that everything is the Tao, everything is the Way. The Tao cannot really be likened to our Western concept of God, more to an idea of cosmic energy – without form or substance but all-powerful and all-pervading.

From the Tao, the Way, comes everything in the known universe. According to Taoists everything can be divided into Heaven and Creation, or spirit and matter. Heaven is represented as a circle and creation, sitting in the middle of heaven, as a square.

Yin and yang

From heaven, spirit, the circle was reduced to an unbroken line called *yang*, while creation, matter, became a broken line called *yin*. The yin/yang symbolism was further developed into the most well-known of all Chinese symbols, shown in figure 1.1.

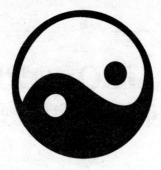

Fig. 1.1 The yin–yang symbol

This is sometimes known as the T'ai Ch'i, the Supreme Ultimate or the Great Art. From the Supreme Ultimate there comes the Tao. From the Tao comes yang and yin and from those two opposites there is everything in balance. Although the yang and yin are sometimes seen as opposites by Westerners within each there is always an element of the other. This is why there is always the tiny dot of white within the black yin, and the tiny dot of dark within the white of the yang.

	Yin	Yang
The world		
	female	male
	receptive	creative
	dark	light
	night	day
	cold	heat
	soft	hard
	wet	dry
	winter	summer
	shadow	sunshine
	inner	outer
	down	up
	north	south
	matter	spirit
	creation	heaven
	earth	sky
	negative	positive
	passive	active

The body

interior	surface
abdomen	back
chest	spine
blood	ch'i energy
cloudy body fluids	clear body fluids

The disease

retiring	advancing
lingering	hasty
weak	powerful
decaying	flourishing
patient feels cold	patient feels hot
skin cold to touch	skin hot to touch
low temperature	high temperature
shivering	feverish
chronic	acute
non-active	virulent
moist	dry

This list is by no means exhaustive: the Chinese classify everything in heaven and earth as either yin or yang. The problem most Westerners have with this is that they tend to see yin and yang as opposites, two extremes; something is yin/female or something is yang/male. The Chinese, however, are always aware of the seed of the yang in the yin and the seed of the yin in the yang: nothing is ever only one or the other, there is always a balance within the thing itself.

The yin/yang symbol can be used to represent the human body, with the head at the top representing spirit – yang, and the body below representing matter – yin. The left-hand side of the body is yang; the right-hand side is yin. (See figure 1.2.)

The beginning of life originates from yin/yang. Yin grows from yang, yang grows from yin and neither can exist without the other. Illness can be seen as resulting from an imbalance of the two.

The abilities of the human body are seen as yang, while food, the energy source, is seen as yin. The body depends on food for life and yet to obtain the energy from the food it must act on it, by digesting it. Too much or too little food can result in excessive or insufficient yang.

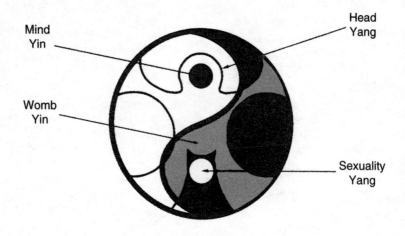

Mind
Yin

Womb
Yin

Head
Yang

Sexuality
Yang

Figure 1.2 Yin/yang with human body

The various organs and systems of the human body are constantly active and so energy is constantly being needed and depleted. Too much need or too much depletion can both result in illness. For example a weakening of yin and an over-expansion of yang could result in high blood-pressure with the symptoms of dizziness, headache, short temper, sleeplessness, irritability, a tight pulse which is slower than normal and a red-coloured tongue.

The seasons and directions

The yin/yang symbol should always be shown with the yin dot to the right. This begins to give us compass directions (see figure 1.3). The light yang is at the top representing summer and the south, while the dark yin is at the bottom representing winter and the north. Chinese compasses are the opposite way round to those in the West: they have their south at the top where our north would be, and their west to the right and east to the left.

We can combine the yin north and yang south to create another two symbols to represent east and west, spring and autumn. (See figure 1.4.)

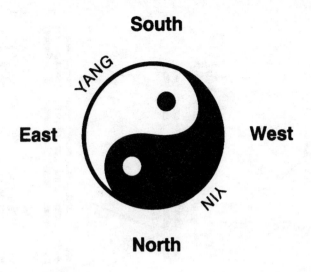

Figure 1.3 Yin/yang with compass directions

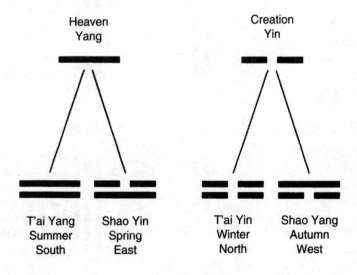

Figure 1.4 The two lines

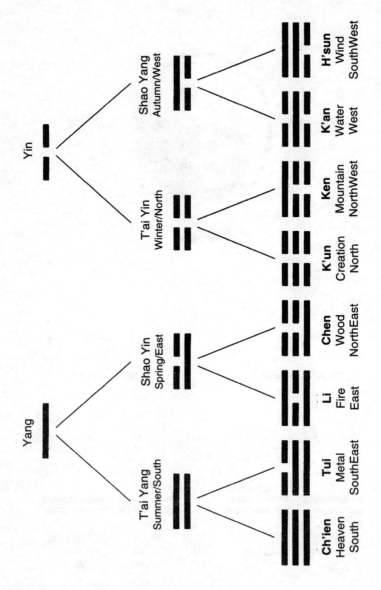

Figure 1.5 The Eight Trigrams

From these four new symbols we can then produce another four to give us the rest of the compass and the mid-season points. (See figure 1.5.)

These are known as the eight trigrams (a trigram consists of three parallel lines). The top lines represent the duality of heaven and creation – the yin/yang. The middle lines represent heaven and creation coming together to create the four seasons and the cardinal points of the compass. The bottom lines represent us, people.

The eight trigrams are all named and have various significance and attributes. They are listed below along with their Chinese name and its translation, their seasons, direction and main attributes.

- Ch'ien – The Creative, heaven, south, summer
- Tui – The Lake, metal, south-east, joy
- Li – The Clinging, fire, east, spring, the sun
- Chen – The Arousing, wood, north-east, thunder
- K'un – The Receptive, creation, north, winter
- Ken – The Stillness, mountain, north-west,
- K'an – The Dangerous, water, west, autumn, the moon
- H'sun – The Wind, gentle, south-west, wood.

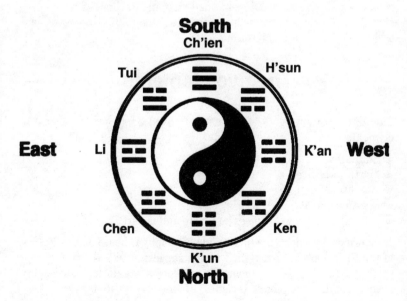

Figure 1.6 The Pah Kwa, the Great Symbol (Former Heaven Sequence)

We can now form these trigrams into an octagon to give us the compass and the seasons (see figure 1.6.). This is known as the Pah Kwa, the Great Symbol, a powerful symbol for the Chinese, representing as it does almost all their spiritual and philosophical beliefs in one image.

The eight trigrams are thought to have been developed by Emperor Fu Hsi around 3000 BC. It is said that he found the eight trigrams in the ornate markings on the shell of a tortoise which he studied on the banks of the Yellow River. The sequence in which he found them is known as the Former Heaven Sequence because around 1000 BC they were rearranged into a different sequence called the Later Heaven Sequence by King Wen, a philosopher and founder of the Chou Dynasty.

The I Ching

These eight trigrams can be paired into 64 new symbols (8 × 8) called hexagrams, which use six lines. These 64 hexagrams each have a meaning; Fu Hsi used them first as a herbal and agricultural almanac which he called the *I Ching* (pronounce: *ee ching*), the Book of Changes. As this was over 5,000 years ago the *I Ching* is probably the oldest book in existence and it has remained virtually unchanged to the present day. The only major restructuring was done by King Wen, who added to Fu Hsi's interpretations.

The five elements

The four cardinal points of the Later Heaven Sequence are also four elements:

- South/fire/li
- North/water/k'an
- East/wood/chen
- West/metal/tui
- The fifth element occupies the centre and is earth.

Most oriental wisdom, medicine and philosophy is based on the Theory of the Five Aspects (Wu Hsing) which suggests that, whilst we are a combination of all of the elements or aspects, we do tend to display predominantly the characteristics of one over the others. These elements are not those of Western astrology. It is better to regard them more as aspects of character.

- Wood – liver and gall bladder network – is said to regulate the movement of ch'i, store the blood and govern temperament.
- Fire – heart and small intestine network – noted as the Emperor network: and the seat of consciousness (it provides a home for the Shen – life-force) in addition to its role in propelling the blood.
- Earth – spleen – stomach network – manages digestion and fluid equilibrium, generating and distributing nourishment.
- Metal – lung and large intestine network – commands respiration and the defences, receiving and dispersing ch'i.
- Water – kidney, urinary and bladder network – rules reproduction, development, growth and maturation. The kidney generates and stores the *essence* (Jing) and is sometimes referred to as 'the root of life, the well of vitality and endurance'.

Each of the five elements gives its own unique personality to the person, which can be briefly summed up as:

- Wood – Mu – The Pioneer – expansive, purposeful, active, likes to be busy, can be domineering, needs to win, practical, should avoid windy places.
- Fire – Huo – The Magician – compassionate, intuitive, communicative, likes pleasure, seeks excitement, likes to be in love, easily bored, should avoid heat.
- Earth – T'u – The Diplomat – moderate, sense of loyalty, harmonious, likes to belong, pays attention to detail, likes company, needs to be needed, can be stubborn, should avoid damp.
- Metal – Chin – The Catalyst – organised, likes to control, precise, discriminating, needs to be right, likes order and cleanliness, appreciates quality, should avoid dryness.
- Water – Shui – The Philosopher – imaginative, honest, clever, seeks knowledge, original, tough, independent, can be secretive, needs to be protected, should avoid cold.

Knowing which element you are will be helpful in your understanding of Chinese medicine as each of the different elements has contrasting responses to the others:

- Wood helps fire, is helped by water, hinders earth, is hindered by metal.
- Fire helps earth, is helped by wood, hinders metal, is hindered by water.
- Earth helps metal, is helped by fire, hinders water, is hindered by wood.

☻ Metal helps water, is helped by earth, hinders wood, is hindered by fire.

☻ Water helps wood, is helped by metal, hinders fire, is hindered by earth.

Each of these five elements rule or influence different internal organs, parts of the body, emotional expressions, colours, tastes and energies. They are also indicative of very different types of people. For example, wood people tend to be supple, muscular, strong and slim. They may suffer from high blood pressure. They may have vertigo and can be short-tempered, prone to sprained ankles and wrists, tension in neck and across shoulders, migraines and tension headaches, constipation, etc. They tend to be quick, decisive people, restless and impatient. They are usually competitive and impulsive. And their complaints can be easily and quickly recognised by a Chinese doctor and treated accordingly.

	Wood	Fire	Earth	Metal	Water
Zang internal organs	Liver	Heart	Spleen	Lungs	Kidneys
Fu internal organs	Gall bladder	Small intestine	Stomach	Large intestine	Bladder
Facial features	Eyes	Tongue	Mouth	Nose	Ears
Body	Tendons	Pulse	Muscle	Skin/hair	Bones
Expression	Anger	Gaiety	Thought	Worry	Fright
Colour	Green	Red	Yellow	White	Black
Taste	Sour	Bitter	Sweet	Pungent	Salt
Energy	Wind	Hot	Wet	Dry	Cold
Season	Spring	Summer	Late summer	Autumn	Winter
Smell	Rancid	Scorched	Fragrant	Putrid	Rotten
Direction	East	South	Centre	West	North

Elemental rulerships

This grouping is known as Five Phase Theory. From this arises the Harmony of the Five Sentiments, these being anger, joy, fear, sorrow, and pensiveness, giving a total of a basic 25 combinations. To keep the body healthy it is necessary to keep these sentiments in balance.

-The Harmony of the Five Sentiments -

Anger

If the emotion of anger dominates then the patient will be easily upset by frustrations, prone to give in to violent outbursts, be volatile and unpredictable. They can be seen by others as self-controlled and self-disciplined but when stress and tension build up they can explode into rage. They are prone to ulcers, migraines and haemorrhoids.

Joy

When joy is the main motivating force in a person's life they are liable to suffer extreme mood swings: they're either up or down, never in between. They can become endless 'pleasure seekers'. They crave excitement and feel empty and alone without it. They are prone to anorexia, schizophrenia, manic-depressive psychosis or hypoglycaemia.

Fear

The person who lives their life with fear can become isolated, hermit-like, even withdrawn. They anticipate the worst, imagine the worst-case scenario in everything they do. They cut themselves off from the world believing it to be a fundamentally evil place which is out to harm them. They are prone to deafness, arthritis and senility.

Sorrow

This person will isolate themselves from excitement or any emotional activity to protect themselves from the emotion they fear most: sorrow. They believe that is what they deserve and subsequently shut off from the world of relationships. They like to control everyone around them so no one can hurt them. Possible illnesses are constipation, frigidity and asthma.

Pensiveness

This patient basically worries over little details to the point of obsession. They get bogged down in minutiae. They like security and safety and can become lethargic and apathetic when faced with new challenges mainly because it is all too much for them. Illnesses tend to show up as obesity, poor digestion, heart problems and high blood-pressure.

——— Is your cold hot or cold? ———

For a Western doctor it may be sufficient to know that we have influenza, but a Chinese doctor will want to know if your influenza is hot or cold, wet or dry. Even our sweat will be classified as hot or cold. If we suffer from a hot fever our doctor will prescribe a cooling herb to counteract the heat, or use the correct acupuncture point. Similarly if we have a shivering cold we will be treated with a heating herb to warm us, or via a different acupuncture point.

——— The flow of ch'i ———

Chinese philosophy allocates everything its yin or yang qualities and identifies an energy, ch'i, that binds them all together and flows within and around them. Ch'i is one of the four most important aspects of traditional Chinese medicine, the other three being blood, internal organs and meridians. When ch'i flows well there is harmony and balance; when it stagnates it is the cause of many, if not all, illnesses. It can be seen as the underlying principle behind the Tao. Ch'i is the invisible force that animates everything, the life-force. We cannot see, touch, taste, hear or feel it but we are aware of it by its effect. Creation is ch'i taking shape. When we die the living ch'i leaves our bodies.

The way ch'i flows in and around our dwellings is called *feng shui*. Feng shui can be seen as aligning our dwellings and ourselves to receive the maximum benefit of good ch'i.

There are four types of external ch'i:

☯ Sheng ch'i – growing ch'i from the east
☯ Yang ch'i – nourishing ch'i from the south
☯ T'sang ch'i – hidden ch'i from the north
☯ Sha ch'i – disruptive ch'i from the west.

Ch'i is dealt with more fully in the next chapter.

2
CH'I, BLOOD AND BODY FLUIDS

Under these two aspects, it is really the same; but as development takes place, it receives the different names. Together we call them the Mystery. Where the Mystery is the deepest is the gate of all that is subtle and wonderful.

Tao Ti Ching

Ch'i

You should by now have some idea of the connections between the compass directions, yin and yang, and ch'i. When ch'i is disruptive (*sha*) it can cause ill health. Chinese medicine can help correct the imbalance but it may sometimes be necessary to move house completely. Your Chinese doctor will ask many questions at your initial consultation, including where and how you live. This information is useful in helping make a diagnosis as the Chinese know well that nothing works in isolation: we are all connected with everyone and everything else.

In Chinese medicine ch'i is regarded as a yang force, the source of growth, and the prime mover and consolidating force of the blood. It organises the whole body, repels attack from outside and promotes the functioning of the internal organs.

The four types of ch'i

Within the body ch'i is further categorised into four types: Original, Internal organ; Guarding; and Protein. We will now look at each in turn.

Original ch'i

Sometimes known as real or correct ch'i, original ch'i represents the strengths and weaknesses of the body in combating all forms of illness. If the original ch'i is weak, infection can take place: restoring original ch'i will ward off illness.

Internal organ ch'i

This is the specific energy of particular organs: there is liver ch'i, heart ch'i, lungs ch'i and so on. The combined ch'i of the stomach and spleen is known as central ch'i. If this becomes weakened it causes difficulties in the function of the digestive system, a slowing down in the rate of mental activity, weak voice and problems with the uterus. These conditions must be treated by a method which strengthens central ch'i.

The ch'i of the lungs and heart together is known as 'ancestral ch'i' and assists respiration and circulation. If the ancestral ch'i is weakened it causes a weak heartbeat and problems with breathing.

Guarding ch'i

This surrounds all the meridians and is dispersed throughout the whole body. It travels outside the meridians and is regarded as the boundary fence of all internal systems.

Protein ch'i

This ch'i travels within the pulse meridians and provides vital protein to the blood and it can be seen that guarding ch'i and protein ch'i work very closely together: the outer and the inner.

The disruption of ch'i

Ch'i can be disrupted in one of three ways: weakening, stagnation or mischannelling.

Weakening ch'i

This means that there is insufficient energy. This is most commonly noticeable when the ch'i of the lungs and the spleen is weakened. The symptoms of this are a loss of appetite, reluctance to speak, sweating for no apparent reason, dizzy spells and a feeble pulse.

Stagnation of ch'i

This occurs when the mechanism of internal organ functioning meets an obstruction to its normal operation, and is found mainly in the spleen, lungs and liver. Stagnation of ch'i in the lungs results in tightness of the chest, pain, wheezy breathing and too much phlegm. Symptoms can include a tightness in the chest, sides and abdomen, accompanied by pain. Ch'i stagnating in the liver produces a bloated abdomen, abdominal pain and a painful and irregular menstrual cycle. Stagnant spleen ch'i produces indigestion and a painful swollen abdomen. Stagnation of ch'i in the meridian veins will result in aching in the muscles and joints of all of the limbs, sometimes with swelling.

Mischannelling of ch'i

This takes place when the ch'i flows in the wrong direction. Each organ's ch'i flows in a particular direction. The stomach and lung ch'i flows downwards and if either flows upwards then illness can result. For example: downward-flowing lung ch'i being reversed would cause asthma and coughs whereas downward-flowing stomach ch'i being reversed would cause vomiting and nausea. Reversed liver ch'i would cause vomiting of blood, fainting and unconsciousness.

Chinese calligraphy and ch'i

The Chinese character for ch'i is a combination of two basic characters. The bottom one is *mi*, which means grains. The original calligraphy depicted four grains. The modern characters look quite similar, but the curved strokes don't look as much like grains. On top of the picture of grains is a calligraphic representation of curling mist rising from the ground and forming clouds above. The curling mist presents the same basic meaning as the yin half that goes into making yin/yang symbol – combining vapours and clouds.

The combined calligraphic representation for ch'i is described as the steam rising from boiling grains (usually rice in the south, millet in the north). But why should this steam from a cooking pot be of sufficient significance to have its own Chinese character, and for this character to be adopted for one of the most important aspects of Chinese medicine? It's probable that the development in food and cooking pots in ancient China made this especially important. Grains, especially rice, are a most important part of Chinese diet. The character for eating (*ch'i*) comes from a picture of a bowl of cooked rice with a spoon.

As the symbols evolved, a new kind of pot was becoming widely used, a bronze cooking pot that had a cover for boiling or steaming of rice in the same way as it is still cooked today. It is probable that rice steam (or grain steam) represented the steam produced in a closed vessel when cooking any food, and was important because it was a very useful means of cooking the most fundamental staple diet of the Chinese.

Ch'i, or food, then becomes representative of the energy explained in Chinese medicine. An early text – the *Gu Jin Yi Tong Da Chuan* (1556) – says: 'Just as fish live in water, humans live in ch'i. If the water is stagnant, the fish waste away. If the ch'i noxious, we suffer ill health.' You might say that as a fish lives in water, we live in air; if the water is polluted the fish die, if the air is polluted, we fall ill. You might assume that ch'i is air, as many people have done; even translating ch'i as air and comparing it to the Indian term *prana*. But ch'i is not air.

Positive and negative ch'i

Ch'i is capable of becoming poisonous despite the fact that the air may be breathable and clean and fresh. The causes of ill health were attributed to failing ch'i, which was thought to be caused by six atmospheric conditions: wind, cold, heat, summer heat (humidity), damp and dryness. Ch'i is thus seen as an influence – one which can be positive or negative. Negative, or obnoxious, ch'i is called *sha*. Just as the steam from a cooking pot has positive qualities – it cooks your food – so it also has negative qualities – it burns you if you put your hand into it. The steam can be seen to continue its upward journey and become clouds which bring positive rain; but too much rain causes flooding, which is a negative quality. Everything in the universe can be see in this twofold way – both positive and negative. Too much or too little of anything becomes negative. Chinese medicine strives to find the right balance – just the right amount to bring good health. Ch'i itself can be excessive within the human body. Normally, this ch'i nourishes the organs, but if it becomes excessive it has a negative effect. The internal ch'i is said to come from food.

In Chinese medicine the human stomach is often described as the 'cooking pot'. When food enters the stomach, it gets heated (cooked) and ch'i gets generated just as ch'i gets generated by cooking rice in a pot. In order for this process to proceed, there must be a cooking fire. In the body, this is the fire of the kidney (of the right kidney, or *mingmen* – vital gate). Just as you have a fire, a cooking pot, rice, and rice steam in cooking, so too in the body you have the kidney fire, the stomach cooking pot, the eaten rice, and the rice-steam (ch'i).

The ch'i from the stomach is said to rise up first to the lungs. The lungs are described as being like a cloud in the heavens, which then rains down the ch'i to the other organs. Just as you have mists rising from the earth, forming clouds in the sky, and then raining down, you have the ch'i rising from the stomach (associated with the earth element in the Five Element Theory) up to the lungs, where it condenses to form the raining clouds. The rain filters down into the water courses (in the body, these are dominated by the organ of the water element, the kidneys).

You may even wonder why it is said that metal helps or produces water, which is not something we'd usually associate with metal. However, if you remember those bronze cooking pots and how important they were to the Chinese just as their culture and concepts were developing, you can see that the metal pot does something that was not done by previous cooking methods: the water is condensed and recirculated. Just as the steam rises from the water-rice mixture and condenses (appears to be produced) on the metal cover of the cooking pot, so the ch'i rises from the eaten rice and condenses in the lungs, which are represented by the metal element.

If we look at the notion of ch'i being energy or steam rising from the cooking rice we can see how the concept of yin and yang can evolve. Yin is the solid matter, the process of condensation from the earth below, whereas yang is the condensation, the mist or steam rising up to the clear sky above. According to Taoist philosophers, in the beginning there is the void, and, either the void is truly empty and gives rise to ch'i, or the void is full of formless ch'i. Then there is a duality; the yin (earth) and yang (heaven). Similarly, in the body, food is separated into the solid and liquid aspects.

Blood

Whereas ch'i is seen as yang, blood is seen as yin: the two providing a nourishing balance and complementing each other. They are both equally necessary for a healthy body. An old Chinese saying is: 'Blood gives birth to ch'i, but ch'i rules the blood.' The motivating energy of ch'i encourages the blood to flow. If the ch'i stagnates, the blood clots.

If there is an inadequate supply of blood a loss of sensitivity and even paralysis can result.

Illnesses related to the blood can be divided into three main categories: escape, weakness and clotting. These are dealt with below.

Escape of the blood

Blood escaping from any of the major organs can be caused by a number of factors which would have to be examined independently. The vomiting of blood, for example, would be seen very differently from excessive menstrual bleeding. Normal bleeding from cuts and wounds would not be seen as escape of the blood but as injuries.

Weakness of the blood

Symptoms of weak blood can include: pallor of the lips, yellowish colour of the skin, pale tongue and nails, blurred sight, dizziness, fainting spells and exhaustion. Anaemia is one example of this. Restoring ch'i can strengthen the blood. If there has been a heavy loss of blood then the body's natural ability to manufacture blood may be impaired. Blood transfusions are a new idea in China as they have always regarded blood as precious and not something to be given away.

Clotting of blood

Ch'i stagnating can cause blood to clot; if this occurs in the lungs then the patient may well cough up blood. Clotting is most commonly seen in the form of bruising, which is usually treated by simple massage or cold-water massage. Ice can be used to good effect to relieve bruising.

Blood clotting may be caused by external bleeding and can develop in the veins of the heart. It can also occur in the limbs or lungs and can be very painful, affecting movement.

Body fluids

In Chinese medicine spirit has two meanings. It is a term for the vital force of the cells which is required for human growth but it also means sperm. Spirit is normally seen as being stored in the kidneys, a part of which, the Chinese believe, becomes sperm.

Juices and dew

All body fluids, even tears and sweat, are categorised as either juices or dew. The fluid dispersed between the joints and in the brain is known as juices; that dispersed among the internal organs, skin and muscles is dew.

Blood and dew are seen as closely related, even thought of as coming from one source, and patients with a blood loss condition would never be treated with a sudorific (medicine to promote sweating).

Phlegm is a form of dew which the Chinese say is developed in the spleen and stored in the lungs. When excessive phlegm is produced in the lungs in such conditions as asthma it cannot settle properly. A remedy would be prescribed that would either disperse or expel the phlegm.

As you may begin to see, the holistic view of Chinese practitioners is that everything is linked, everything inter-dependent on everything else within the human body. Even the outside of the body is regarded as yang while the inside is yin. Life and death are seen as yang while birth and growth are yin. The Chinese herbal practitioner strives always to restore the balance, the harmony, between yin and yang and knows that each change will subtly alter other parts of the human body.

3
PREVENTATIVE
MEDICINE

*The Tao is (like) the emptiness of a vessel; and in our
employment of it we must be on our guard against all fullness. How
deep and unfathomable it is, as if it were the Honoured Ancestor of
all things!*

Tao Ti Ching

Ch'i Kung

Ch'i Kung (pronounced *chee goong*, and you may see it spelt as:
qi gong) is a Chinese system of physical training, philosophy, and preventative and therapeutic health care. *Ch'i* (or *qi*) means air, breath
of life, energy or vital essence. *Kung* means work, self-discipline,
achievement or mastery. This art combines aerobic conditioning, iso-
metrics, isotonics, meditation, and relaxation. Ch'i Kung is a discipline whose practice allows us to gain control over the life-force that
courses through our bodies. There are more than 3,000 varieties of
Ch'i Kung, and five major Ch'i Kung traditions: the Taoist, Buddhist,
Confucian, martial arts, and medical. Ch'i Kung is a soft form of a
related set of disciplines that includes Tai Ch'i (Tai Ch'i Chuan) and
the hard form of Kung Fu.

Like the other forms, medical Ch'i Kung involves the cultivation and
control of ch'i. It is a system of exercises, involving breathing and
meditation, which improve health and longevity as well as increasing
the sense of harmony within oneself and in the world. There are
thousands of such exercises. In fact, anything you do with the intention of benefiting your energy can be considered Ch'i Kung. All Ch'i

Kung contains common principles – mind, eyes, movement and breath. People of all ages can learn to practise Ch'i Kung, and so develop and maintain internal vigour and good health.

The history of Ch'i Kung

The history of Chinese Ch'i Kung can be roughly divided into four periods. Little is known about the first period, which is considered to have started when the *I Ching* (Book of Changes) was introduced sometime before 1122 BC, and to have extended until the Han dynasty (206 BC) when Buddhism and its meditation methods were imported from India. This intermingling brought Ch'i Kung practice and meditation into the second period, the religious Ch'i Kung era. This period lasted until the Liang dynasty (AD 502–7), when it was discovered that Ch'i Kung could be used for martial purposes. This was the beginning of the third period, that of martial Ch'i Kung. Many different martial Ch'i Kung styles were created based on the theories and principles of Buddhist and Taoist Ch'i Kung. This period lasted until the overthrow of the Ch'ing dynasty in 1911; from that point Chinese Ch'i Kung training was mixed with Ch'i Kung practices from India, Japan, and many other countries.

During the Cultural Revolution (1965–76) the Communist Party and Red Guards suppressed Ch'i Kung. In about 1978 it began to make a comeback. In the 1980s there was an upsurge of interest in Ch'i Kung in China. Today more than 70 million Chinese practise it every day. Some do this to treat and cure an existing illness; others are trying to prevent the onset of disease; still others want to feel and perform better, experience higher levels of energy and stamina, and slow down the ageing process.

Ch'i Kung is rapidly spreading throughout North America and the rest of the Western world. In 1988 the Chinese held in Beijing the first World Conference for exchanging Ch'i Kung medical research. And since then world conferences have taken place in Tokyo and Berkeley. Another took place in the summer of 1996 in New York City. Today, North American psychological, physiological and medical researchers are studying Ch'i Kung with increasing interest, and there are many Ch'i Kung websites on the Internet.

The Chinese have found Ch'i Kung an effective way to treat drug and alcohol abuse and obesity. This gentle art improves delivery of oxygen to the body's cells, reduces stress and improves bowel functioning.

Chinese doctors have applied Ch'i Kung in hospitals and clinics to treat individuals suffering from a variety of ailments. These include allergies, arthritis, asthma, bowel problems, constipation, diabetes, gastritis, gout, headaches, heart disease and hypertension; chronic kidney disease, liver disease, lower back pain, Meniere's disease, myopia, obesity, neurasthenia, paralysis induced by external injury, retinopathy (deterioration of the back of the eye), rheumatism, sciatic neuralgia, sleeplessness, stress, torticollis, ulcers, and peripheral vascular disease.

Ch'i Kung has been used successfully to treat cancer and also to reduce or eliminate side-effects from radiation and chemotherapy. It is helpful in treating aphasia (loss or impairment of ability to speak), cerebral palsy, multiple sclerosis, Parkinson's disease and post-stroke syndrome. It is especially useful in treating any kind of chronic pain, and chronic disorders of the digestive, respiratory, cardiovascular and nervous systems.

Ch'i Kung can help one fight virtually any disease. Through Ch'i Kung, patients can cure many of the diseases that Western doctors dismiss as untreatable. However, curative Ch'i Kung should only be carried out under the supervision of a qualified Chinese medicine practitioner.

Avoiding disease

Ch'i Kung is most effective in treating chronic illness and preventing the onset of disease. This can save money and prevent suffering. Ch'i Kung increases strength, improves resistance to infectious diseases and premature senility, and helps assure a long life. Practising Ch'i Kung can greatly reduce the danger of stroke. It can improve blood sugar levels for diabetics. Because it normalises the level of sex hormones, it can correct sexual impotence and frigidity. Its stress-relieving effects improve one's sex life – both quantity and quality. Practice of Ch'i Kung can speed recovery from surgery, and from sports and other injuries by up to 50 per cent.

Ch'i Kung offers individuals a way to achieve a relaxed, harmonious state of dynamic equilibrium. It typically improves their overall health status, allowing them to maintain a life free from pain, and full of vigour and grace. Ch'i Kung is a proper therapeutic practice with which to address virtually any chronic health problem. The various forms of Chinese medical massage (Tui Na) derive directly from Ch'i

Kung. These practices compliment and supplement orthodox medical interventions.

Chinese herbal medicine, acupuncture, and Ch'i Kung are three parts of a single medical practice. They can be used separately or together. With dietetics and massage they are considered to be the indispensable components of traditional Chinese health care. While acupuncture and herbal medicine typically focus on curing sickness, Ch'i Kung usually focuses on maintaining good health (as do massage and balanced nutrition).

In the philosophy of Ch'i Kung, a primary aim is to maintain or restore balance and harmony of mind and body. Through Ch'i Kung, you can build up ch'i and move it to where a disturbance or blockage occurs.

Ch'i Kung lowers blood-pressure, pulse rates, metabolic rates, lactate production and oxygen demand. The sense of serenity Ch'i Kung produces results partly from a slightly increased body temperature, and an increased rate of oxygen absorption. Ch'i Kung activates ch'i, improves blood circulation, and balances yin and yang. It bolsters the immune system, and stimulates the conductivity of the meridians and channels through which ch'i flows. When the immune system is strong, when one is emotionally centred within one's body, and when ch'i and blood are flowing freely, then most diseases should disappear.

The goal of practising Ch'i Kung is to make the ch'i circulate well in the body. This helps us resist or overcome imbalances or blockages and their resulting disharmonies. That is also the goal of acupuncture and Chinese herbal medicine. Chinese medicine can prolong life, vitality and well-being by slowing the ageing process. This it accomplishes due to the affinities of certain herbs to ch'i and the environment within which ch'i exists. Ch'i Kung therefore 'fits' into the regimen of Chinese medicine.

One need not become a Ch'i Kung practitioner to experience many of its healing effects. For health purposes, you need to learn only a few exercises. Conversely, Ch'i Kung is far from being an instant cure-all. To benefit through personal effort alone one must achieve a state of tranquillity, find release from tension, build a positive attitude, and develop strong, committed will-power. There are three ways to benefit from Ch'i Kung. First, one can go to a practitioner for treatment by that practitioner's external ch'i. Second, one can seek treatment from a practitioner and practise exercise and meditation. Thirdly, one can learn to treat oneself. To gain full benefits of Ch'i Kung through self-treatment requires time, patience, commitment to its practice, determination and persistence. This art involves more than simple physical training. It requires educating your breathing and thought processes. This means increasing your ability to sense your body, and to feel and imagine. As with any other aspect of human endeavour, some people will prove more adept at the art than others, and so will progress more quickly. However, anyone with enough motivation can learn adequate Ch'i Kung skills to make a large impact upon their life. This can take from a minimum of three months up to a year. There are no shortcuts. There are also, though, no obvious limits to how far one may progress.

Because Ch'i Kung thins blood and increases circulation, women should not practise it during menstruation. If you have internal bleeding, or bleeding after tooth extraction or trauma, avoid Ch'i Kung exercises until the condition disappears. Avoid exercising if you feel dizzy. Ch'i Kung is not for severely disturbed mental patients, pregnant women or people suffering from acute infectious diseases. Avoid food and drink for an hour and a half before a session. Especially avoid alcohol. When exercising, face either north or south, in line with the earth's magnetic field. Exercise at the same time(s) of day and the same days through the week. Avoid sexual intercourse for at least one hour before and after a Ch'i Kung session.

There are limits to what you can learn about Ch'i Kung from reading. One really should begin to practise this art by enrolling in a course or joining an organised group.

Basic rules for Ch'i Kung practice

☯ Be patient
  When you take up Ch'i Kung you are enthusiastic and eager.
  However, sometimes you don't learn as fast as you would like to, and
  you could become impatient and try to force things. This is not helpful.
☯ Regulate your sexual activity
  You should not have sexual relations at least an hour before or
  after practising Ch'i Kung, 24 hours in the case of martial, religious
  or healing Ch'i Kung. Sex depletes your Ch'i and sperm, and the
  Ch'i level in the lower portion of your body is lower than normal.
☯ Keep the temperature even
  The temperature of the room in which you are training should not
  be too hot or too cold. You should practise in the most comfortable
  place possible.

☙ Be careful of the Five Weaknesses and internal injuries
Five weaknesses means the weaknesses of five yin organs: the
heart, liver, lungs, kidneys, and spleen. When you realise that any
of these five organs is weak, you should proceed very gradually and
gently with your Ch'i Kung practice. Ch'i Kung practice is an
internal exercise which is directly related to these five organs.
For the same reason, when you have an internal injury your
internal Ch'i distribution and circulation is already disturbed. If
you practise Ch'i Kung your feelings may be misled, and your
practice may worsen your problem and interfere with the natural
healing process.

☙ Avoid breezes when sweating
Don't practise in the wind, especially facing the wind. When you
practise Ch'i Kung you are exercising either internally, or both
internally and externally. It is normal to sweat, and since you are
relaxed, your pores are wide open. If you expose your body to cold
wind, you will catch cold.

☙ Wear loose clothing
Always wear loose clothes during practice because this will help
you to feel comfortable. Keep your belt loose, too. The abdomen is
the key area in Ch'i Kung practice, and you must be careful not to
limit the movement of this area because it will interfere with your
practice.

☙ Watch what you eat
You should regulate your eating habits while you are practising
Ch'i Kung. Too much rich or sweet food will increase your fire ch'i,
which can confuse the mind. You should eat more fruit and
vegetables, and avoid alcohol and tobacco.

☙ Wear clean dry clothing
When your clothes are wet from sweat you will feel uncomfortable,
and your concentration will be affected. It is better to change into
dry clothes and then resume practice.

☙ Don't practise on a full stomach
You should not practise Ch'i Kung when hungry or when your
stomach is full. When you are hungry it is hard to concentrate, and
when you are full your practice will affect your digestion.

☙ Watch the weather
It is believed that your body's ch'i is directly affected by changes in
the weather. It is therefore not advisable to practise Ch'i Kung
when there is a sudden weather change, because your practice will
interfere with your body's natural readjustment to the new
environment. You will also be unable to feel and sense your ch'i

flow as you do normally. You must always try to remain emotionally neutral whenever you do Ch'i Kung. Even if you are disturbed by a natural disaster like an earthquake, you must remain calm so that your ch'i stays under control.

☯ Don't think about what you are doing

When you practise, do not place your attention on the various phenomena or sensations which are occurring. Be aware of what is happening, but keep your mind centred on wherever it is supposed to be for the exercise you are doing. When you drive a car, you don't watch yourself steer and work the pedals and change gear. You simply put your mind on where you want to go and let your body automatically drive the car. This is called regulating without regulating.

☯ Keep a still mind

Keep your thoughts located and focused on what you are doing and don't allow your mind to wander and think about other things.

☯ Be aware of what is happening around you

You should be aware of what is going on around you but don't focus on it. Noises you hear should be ignored, as should body sensations like itches and tickles.

☯ Only practise what has been shown you

You need to have confidence when you practise Ch'i Kung. You should not listen to advice from people who do not have experience in Ch'i Kung and who are not familiar with the condition of your body. Only practise what you have been shown by your Ch'i Kung teacher.

☯ Stay awake

You should not continue your Ch'i Kung training when you are sleepy. When you are sleepy your body will not be regulated and will tend to lean or droop, and your bad posture may interfere with the proper Ch'i circulation. When you are sleepy it is best to take a rest.

☯ Don't practise unless you are calm

You should not meditate when you are too excited due to anger or happiness. Since your mind is scattered, meditation will bring you more harm than peace.

☯ Don't keep spitting

It is normal to generate a lot of saliva while practising Ch'i Kung. The saliva should be swallowed to moisten your throat. Don't spit out the saliva because this is a waste, and it will also disturb your concentration.

☯ Retain your confidence

When you first start Ch'i Kung, you must have confidence in what you are doing, and not start doubting its validity, or questioning whether you are doing it right. If you start doubting right at the beginning you will become lazy, and you will start questioning whether you really want to continue. In this case, you will not have any success and your practice will never last.

☉ Remember that Ch'i Kung takes a long time to learn properly
This is to remind you that Ch'i Kung practice is time-consuming and progress is slow. You must have patience, a strong will, and confidence to reach your goal. Taking it easy and being natural are the most important rules.

☉ Don't hang your feet off the bed
Traditionally the most common place to practise Ch'i Kung was sitting on a bed. Since most beds were high, if you sat on the edge of the bed your feet would hang off the side of the bed above the floor. When you practise Ch'i Kung your feet should touch the floor. If they do not, all of the weight of your body will press down on the lower part of your thighs and reduce the Ch'i and blood circulation. Furthermore, when you practise you should not put your feet up on the table, because this position will also stagnate the Ch'i and blood circulation.

☉ Don't practise with a full bladder
You should go to the toilet before you start your practice. If you need to go during practice, stop and do so. Holding it in disturbs your concentration.

☉ Don't scratch an itch
If you itch because of some external reason, such as an insect walking on you or biting you, do not be alarmed and keep your mind calm. You may scratch or think of how to stop the itching. However, if the itching is caused by ch'i redistribution in the Ch'i Kung practice, remain calm and do not move your mind there. Simply ignore it and let it happen. Once it has reached a new balance, the itching will stop. If you scratch this kind of itch it means that your mind has been disturbed.

☉ Avoid being suddenly disturbed or startled
You should avoid being suddenly disturbed or startled. However, if it does happen, calm down your mind. Most important of all, though, is learning how to regulate your mind when you are disturbed.

☉ Don't judge what is going on inside you
It is very common during practice to suddenly notice something that is going on inside of you. Perhaps you feel ch'i moving for the first time and you feel elated and excited. You have to learn how to be aware of what is going on inside you without getting excited.

Breathing

In Ch'i Kung special attention must be placed on your breathing, and this is one of the major requirements of successful Ch'i Kung practice. Your breathing should be the same as when you are meditating. This means that upon the in-breath, the lower abdomen will fill from the bottom up. If your breathing is incorrect you will get tired very quickly, and get headaches as well.

The tip of the tongue should be just touching the roof of the mouth. Eyes will be either closed, or only opened part-way. This is to make sure you are not disturbed by external influences and are fully relaxed.

You should gently focus your attention on your hands. You may also focus your attention on your whole body. Do not restrict your thoughts to any specific acupuncture points because this may cause the energy to get bogged down in that area and lead to uncomfortable side-effects, including irritability, sleeplessness, and trouble digesting food.

The exercises

After warming up with a little light exercise, you should train in the following postures for five minutes each.

Posture 1

Place feet at shoulder width, with knees bent so that you only see the tips of your big toes as you look down. Keep your lower back straight by tilting the pelvis forward slightly. It is essential that your posture be comfortable. A kink in the back will cause the energy flow to stagnate, and thus cause muscle cramps and lower back pain.

The same requirements for body posture are held throughout the training.

Extend your arms forward, palms down. Your upper arms should form a 45 degree angle relative to both front and sides of your body, as if you are resting your lower arms flat on a table which is at the height of your sternum.

Posture 2

Rotate the palms so that they face the sky.

Posture 3

Rotate the palms inwards so that they face each other.

Posture 4

Roll the arms so that the left palm is on top, facing down, and the right arm rolls down, and the palm winds up facing the left palm. The left palm will be at mid chest height, and the right palm will be at the level of the navel. The palms will be about three inches away from the body in this posture.

Posture 5

Roll the arms in the opposite directions, so that now the right is on top, palm facing down, and the left palm is on the bottom, facing upwards.

Train in these postures every day for six months. After six months you can add these extra exercises to strengthen the ch'i you have built up previously.

Extra exercise 1

From Posture 3, that is the palms facing each other at chest height, slowly exhale (and gently exhale), and bring the palms close to each other, but do not allow them to touch. Do this exercise in place of the plain standing as you have done previously.

Extra exercise 2

From Posture 4, slowly compress your hands towards each other from the top and the bottom, at the same time. Essentially you are doing extra Posture 1, but from a different angle. Do this series of expanding and contracting movements as you do your standing meditation set.

Extra exercise 3

From Posture 5, do the same movements as outlined above.

Basic adjunctive training: leading the ch'i

Place a lit candle level with your mid–chest area. Place one palm about six inches beyond the candle flame. The other hand, on the near side of the flame, will adopt the 'Sword Fingers' posture: index and middle finger pointing outwards, ring and little finger folded into palm. Lead your ch'i to your index and middle fingers by visualising it as a moving stream of energy. After you have felt the ch'i arrive at those areas, transmit it to the flame. Continue for a few minutes then lead the ch'i that is in the candle flame to your far-side hand, and direct it to the Lao gong point of that hand, in the centre of the palm where the ring finger touches when folded in.

Train both sides for a few minutes each day. This will strengthen your focus and your will, and is good training for emitting the ch'i from the fingers.

Healing with Ch'i Kung

The use of Ch'i energy for healing others is referred to as External Ch'i Healing, External Ch'i Kung, or Ch'i Sao. Ch'i energy is directed through the hands or eyes towards the patient. External Ch'i healing is historically one of the main applications of Ch'i energy cultivation. There are numerous levels and depths to this healing ability. Certain healers using externally directed ch'i seem to have better effects with some illnesses than others. It may be that to become an accomplished practitioner you must develop a wide spectrum of abilities and be able to apply them in a variety of types of imbalances in body, emotions, mind, soul and spirit.

Basic healing

After about nine months of training, your energy is strong enough to begin doing minor healing. This can be as a sole method of treatment, or complementing Western/allopathic treatment. You can work on joint pains, headaches, toothaches and sprains. For large areas, you should use a flat palm. To disperse the pain in a large area, direct the ch'i in your hand to flood the area that is painful for the other person. Then when the patient feels the ch'i, you should describe ever-widening, outwards-going, counter-clockwise circles to disperse and sedate the area of its painful influences. For smaller areas, the sword fingers are very useful.

Make sure that you do not treat too many people in one day, as this will tire you out too easily. Also, if a patient starts getting dizzy during treatment hold off until they have recovered.

Pain

When you get hurt, the normal energy flow in your body is disrupted, and this will manifest as pain.

When a person is in pain, this is a physiological manifestation and a message to the body, that certain structural limits have been exceeded, as in a sprain, or dislocation. Energetically speaking the area of pain has either too much energy, and it knows not where to go, or there is too little energy in the area to maintain functional requirements.

Excess and deficiency

Excessive conditions may manifest physically as overly hot, and/or swollen areas, such as is seen in bruises. Physiologically this is due to trauma to the soft tissues, burst capillaries, and the presence of white blood cells which are removing the damaged tissues.

Deficient conditions may manifest physically as cold spots, and/or overly stiff areas, as seen in some joint injuries, such as frozen shoulder syndrome. Physiologically this can be attributed to a decrease in blood flow to the area. Energetically this is due to a restriction of the flow of ch'i to that area. The area will be weak, and not be able to engage in strenuous physical activity.

Treatment of excessive and deficient conditions

Excessive conditions are treated through the reducing technique. This means that the practitioner will direct their flow of ch'i to the painful area and spread the pain out to such a point that it loses its cohesion, and is absorbed by the surrounding tissues. This technique involves starting at the centre of the pained area, and describing ever-widening, outward-going, counter-clockwise circles. Large areas of pain are best treated using the flat palm method, that is with the palm held about two inches from the area, and employing the method described. Draw the circles slowly, until they reach a range of about three inches from the origin of the painful site, and repeat for at least five minutes, or until the patient indicates that their pain has diminished significantly. The patient will sometimes feel a brief increase of the pain as the chaotic energy is being made to move from its stuck position.

Treatment of deficient conditions is done through the strengthening technique, in which energy from the surrounding areas is drawn in to the painful area. This is also done by the flat palm method. Begin at an area about three inches away from the origin of the pain, and describe ever tighter circles, until they arrive at the centre of the pained area. Repeat the process for about five minutes, or until the patient indicates that the pain has decreased.

Other methods

For large painful areas, the flat palm is a preferred method. For small areas, the index and middle finger held together and extended, with the other fingers bent and held close to the palm. An easier way to describe this is the 'peace sign', except the fingers are together, and not separated.

Another method used is the 'Drawing Down' technique. In this you will place your hands to each side of the painful site, and draw the disordered energy down the limb, thereby over-extending the area at which the pain may have an effect. Hold your hands about two inches from the arm as you draw down the limb. As you inhale and return to the top of the arm, make sure you are not in the path of the arm. The goal is to draw the pain out and down the arm, not to push it back up as you repeat the process. For leg injuries, travel down the leg. For mid to low back pain, also travel down the leg. For upper back pains, lead the energy up the back and out the arm on the side where the pain is. For neck and head pains, lead the energy down the arm on the afflicted side.

How the patient can help

The patient's input is of paramount importance. They will be the ones who can best describe what they are feeling as you work on their pains and injuries. They should be encouraged to give you a progress report on what they are feeling as you proceed.

It is easier to treat an injury if the patient comes to you when it is fresh. If there has been a delay, your first treatment will only partially alleviate the pain. The patient will have to come back for a few treatments, and will notice that the pain becomes less and less after each treatment, until it disappears altogether.

Routine effects on the patient

- ☻ An overall relaxation of the body, and deepening of the breath. If the patient is on a massage table, they may even fall asleep.
- ☻ Tingling of the area as you work on it.
- ☻ A heating up of the limb as the energy is projected to it.
- ☻ They may feel the pain get smaller and smaller until it is no longer palpable, or they may feel the pain expand and disintegrate into nothingness.
- ☻ The patient will also feel the pain as it travels down the limb. This

is nothing to worry about as long as all the pain is dispersed or at least greatly reduced by the end of the treatment session.

Side-effects

Some clients have a low tolerance for the energy and they will display the following symptoms:

☻ confusion
☻ nausea
☻ dizziness
☻ heart palpitations
☻ light-headedness
☻ they may suddenly pass out.

If any of the first five happen, stop the treatment immediately, and let them recoup and start again.

Some clients have a high-energy metabolism, and treating them will take a bit longer. Each treatment session may last anywhere from a few minutes to a half hour or more. Be sensible, and don't overextend your capacities. To do so would cause the quality of your healing energy to decrease, and would not benefit the patient.

Tui Na

Tui Na is an oriental bodywork therapy that has been used in China for 2,000 years. It uses the flow of ch'i through the meridians as its basic therapeutic orientation. Through the application of massage and manipulation techniques Tui Na seeks to establish a more harmonious flow of ch'i through the system of channels and collaterals, allowing the body to heal itself naturally.

Tui Na methods include the use of hand techniques to massage the soft tissue (muscles and tendons) of the body, acupressure techniques to directly affect the flow of ch'i, and manipulation techniques to realign the musculo-skeletal and ligamentous relationships (bone-setting). External herbal poultices, compresses, liniments, and salves are also used to enhance the other therapeutic methods.

Tui Na has a variety of different systems that emphasise particular aspects of these therapeutic principles. The main schools in China include: the rolling method school which emphasises soft tissue techniques and specialises in joint injuries and muscle sprains; the one finger pushing method school, which emphasises techniques for acupressure and the treatment of internal diseases; the Nei Kung method school, which emphasises the use of Nei Kung Ch'i energy-generation exercises and specific massage methods for revitalising depleted energy systems; and the bone-setting method school, which emphasises manipulation methods to realign the musculo-skeletal and ligamentous relationships and specialises in joint injuries and nerve pain.

In a typical session, the patient, wearing loose clothing and no shoes, lies on a table or floor mat. The practitioner examines the specific problems of the patient and begins to apply a specific treatment protocol. The major focus of application is upon specific pain sites, acupressure points, energy meridians, and muscles and joints. Advanced Tui Na practitioners may also use Chinese herbs to facilitate quicker healing. Sessions last from 30 minutes to an hour. Depending on the specific problems of the patient, they may return for additional treatments. The patient usually feels relaxed but energised by the treatment.

Tui Na is gaining in popularity and knowledge throughout the Western world as a powerful therapeutic extension of traditional Western massage methods. Tui Na's simplicity and focus on specific problems, rather than a more generalised treatment, make it both an excellent alternative and/or extension of the Swedish-style massage. By utilising treatments of shorter duration, it can be used in a variety of settings, including home, office, clinic or hospital. It is well suited for both the professional massage therapist or the active, health conscious individual.

History

Tui Na dates back to the Shang dynasty of China, 1700 BC. Oracle bones show that Tui Na massage was used to treat children's diseases and digestive complaints in adults. By AD 600 Tui Na was included in the Imperial Medical College as a separate department. Tui Na flourished throughout China until the Ch'ing dynasty, where it was suppressed along with other Chinese cultural arts. Following the Communist revolution, Tui Na was restored along with other traditional medical arts and was included in the creation of the current system of traditional medicine colleges.

Currently, Tui Na is taught as a separate but equal field of study in the major traditional Chinese medical colleges. Tui Na doctors receive the same demanding training as acupuncturists and herbalists and enjoy the same level of professional respect.

What does Tui Na treat?

Tui Na is well suited for the treatment of specific musculo-skeletal disorders and chronic stress-related disorders of the digestive, respiratory and reproductive systems. Effective treatment protocols have been tested in a practical setting. Tui Na is not especially useful for those seeking a mild, sedating and relaxing massage since it tends to be more task-focused than other types of bodywork. Contra-indications include conditions involving fractures, phlebitis, infectious conditions, open wounds, and lesions.

Tai Ch'i

The Chinese characters for Tai Ch'i Chuan can be translated as the 'Supreme Ultimate Force'. The notion of 'supreme ultimate' is often associated with the Chinese concept of yin and yang, the dynamic duality. 'Force' (or, more literally, 'fist') can be thought of here as the means or way of achieving this yin–yang or 'supreme-ultimate' discipline.

Tai Ch'i, as it is practised in the West today, can perhaps best be thought of as a form of yoga and moving meditation combined. There are a number of so-called forms (sometimes also called 'sets') which consist of a sequence of movements. Many of these movements are originally derived from the martial arts (and perhaps even more basically than that, from the natural movements of animals and birds) although the way they are performed in Tai Ch'i is slowly, softly and gracefully with smooth and even transitions between them.

For many practitioners the focus in doing them is not first and foremost martial, but meditative. For others the combat aspects of Tai Ch'i are of considerable interest. One of the avowed aims of Tai Ch'i is to foster the circulation of ch'i within the body, the belief being that by doing so the health and vitality of the person are enhanced. Ch'i circulates in patterns that are closely related to the nervous and vascular system and thus the notion is closely connected with that of the practice of acupuncture and other oriental healing arts.

Another aim of Tai Ch'i is to foster a calm and tranquil mind, focused on the precise carrying out of these exercises. Learning to do them correctly provides a practical avenue for learning about balance and control. The practice of Tai Ch'i can in some measure contribute to better posture and movement in other spheres of life as well. Many practitioners notice benefits in terms of correcting poor postural, alignment or movement patterns which can contribute to tension or injury. Furthermore the meditative nature of the exercises is calming and relaxing in itself.

Because the Tai Ch'i movements have their origins in the martial arts, practising them does have some martial applications. A two-person exercise called 'push-hands' develops the Tai Ch'i principles of sensitivity and responsiveness to another person's ch'i, or vital energy. It is also an opportunity to employ some of the martial aspects of Tai Ch'i in a kind of slow-tempo combat. Long-time practitioners of Tai Ch'i who are so inclined can become very adept at martial arts. The emphasis in Tai Ch'i is on being able to channel potentially destructive energy (in the form of a kick or a punch) away from one in a manner that will dissipate the energy or send it in a direction where it is no longer a danger.

4

CHINESE HERBAL MEDICINE

*It is better to leave a vessel unfilled, than to attempt to
carry it when it is full. If you keep feeling a point that has been
sharpened, the point cannot long preserve its sharpness.*

Tao Ti Ching

Herbal medicine is itself a powerful method of healing. Western drugs
often control symptoms, but do not alter the disease process (antibiotics eliminate bacteria but do not improve a person's resistance to
infection; diuretics rid excess fluid without improving kidney function). Chinese herbs treat the underlying condition as defined by traditional diagnosis, and rarely cause unwanted side-effects.

Just as soil becomes depleted through overuse, so the ch'i, moisture,
and blood are eroded by overwork, emotional tension, mental strain,
too much or too little exercise, and inadequate diet or rest, impairing
the capacity of the organ networks to do their jobs.

How herbs work

Since fatigue results from a lack of ch'i, herbs that nourish the ch'i
have an energising effect. Since blurry vision, restless sleep and irritability result from depleted blood, blood-enriching herbs improve
vision, sleep, and equanimity. Since dry skin and dehydration arise
from insufficient moisture, herbs that replenish it soften the skin and
relieve an otherwise unquenchable thirst.

Herbs assist the organ networks in the performance of their tasks. Particular herbs enhance the capacity of the heart to propel the blood to soothe the mind, the spleen to manage digestion and fluid equilibrium, the lungs to handle respiration and the body's defences, the liver to maintain resilient emotions and supple limbs, and the kidney to sustain sexual and regenerative power. Some herbal formulas address ailments such as colds, allergies, inflammations or cramps with dramatic and immediate results, while others fortify body reserves over time.

Combination formulas

Chinese herbs are usually combined in formulas to enhance their individual properties and actions. Symptoms and signs are matched with therapeutic effects, reflecting the particular conditions and needs of each patient. Tonic formulas restore eroded body resources; regulating formulas decongest the ch'i, moisture and blood, relieving discomfort; and purging formulas eliminate adverse climates, inviting clear weather.

—— Sources and preparation ——

Obtaining herbs

In China the herbs used are gathered from the wild by hand. The best herbs grow far from human habitation and the herbalist will also be a botanist, explorer, climber and environmentalist; being able to identify the relevant herb in all stages of its development, knowing where the best ones grow, being able to get to them even though they may grow in the wildest most inaccessible places, knowing how much they can take without threatening a particular species and always being on the look-out for new sources and new species. Luckily in the West we can just go to our Chinese herbalist's shop and buy them over the counter.

Most herbs are imported from Hong Kong, although some do come from mainland China via Beijing and Shanghai. Increasingly, as China opens its doors to the West, better access will be granted for importing herbs, but currently the best stocks come from Hong Kong. Some herbalists import their herbs directly while others purchase theirs from Chinese herbal 'cash and carry' stores in the West or from mail order suppliers (see listing at the back of book).

Preservation of herbs

Once the herbs have been collected from the wild they need to be treated to preserve their qualities for storage. They are always washed and dried. The method of drying varies depending on the herb and what it is going to be used for. They may be sun-dried or dried in a clay oven, alone or with other herbs. Sometimes they are dried with minerals such as sulphur, which bleaches them and also acts as a preservative.

Sometimes you will hear of herbs being 'treated'. This means that after drying they are stir-fried with angelica and milk vetch to enhance their properties. Some may also be buried in the ground to absorb moisture or cooked in a clay pot with rice wine or honey to increase their potency.

Cutting up and storage

Before or after they have been dried they will need to be cut up; when this is done depends on the herb and its eventual usage. There are several different ways of cutting herbs. Large roots are often sliced across at 90 degrees, which gives them a round cross section. Smaller herbs are cut at an angle to give a larger surface area. Some herbs are chopped very finely and compressed into a cake.

Traditionally herbs would be stored in clay pots after preservation and cutting up. The shape of the clay pots and whether they were covered or uncovered depended on the herbs. The Chinese have always used clay pots because clay was the simplest and cheapest material to get hold of and also because when glazed the clay, being non-absorbent, helps keep the properties of the herbs intact.

Modern herbalists increasingly use glass jars and bottles for herb storage but still rely on wooden drawers for the bulk of their stocks because it is the easiest and most convenient method of dispensing them. These drawers are rarely labelled, as the herbalist is completely familiar with their contents. Since the drawers are arranged according to meridians and properties it would be hard for the herbalist to make a mistake that would result in a herb of a totally different type being dispensed.

However the herbs are stored the herbalist will check them periodically for mould and or other signs of decay. You don't have to worry about whether these checks will be carried out by your herbalist or not: they will because any fungal infection in any herb is likely to affect their entire stock of herbs. It is in their own best interests to check most of their stocks every day.

Herbs may need to be retreated – washed and boiled, redried and, where necessary, treated with angelica again in the same way that fresh herbs are. When seeds are prescribed they are usually ground using a mortar and pestle. It is said that you can tell who a herbalist is from the sound of their mortar and pestle and they will be judged on their experience and skill by that sound.

Quality

The herbalist will select herbs of a particular quality according to how much money the patient can spend. Different grades of herbs are common. Some herbs from some areas in China are considered superior to the same herb from another area. One herb often graded in this way is ginseng.

Weighing herbs

Because it is so expensive, ginseng is weighed in very sensitive scales which have divisions of 0.1 of a gram. Other herbs do not need quite such accurate scales and larger ones can be used. These are accurate to within approximately 3 grams. Both sorts of scales are used by holding one of the strings near the pan and adjusting the weight on the rod.

Metric weights have been used throughout this book but the Chinese herbalist will use Chinese weights. Their names and approximate metric equivalents are given below.

1 fan		= 0.3 g
10 fan	= 1 qin	= 3 g
10 qin	= 1 lian	= 30 g
16 lian	= 1 jin	= 480 g

Whatever scales are used the weight given is always that of the herb before any stir-frying specified on the prescription. The herbs may be fried in honey, water, or rice wine, or 'burned' until black in a red-hot wok. These treatments naturally change the weight of the herb and it is not unknown for patients to weigh their herbs afterwards and mistakenly complain that they have been short-changed by the herbalist.

Some herbs quite often have to be ground to a powder and this is done using a different type of mortar and pestle: one with a lid to avoid the loss of powder during crushing.

Boiling and steaming

Herbs are boiled in clay pots that naturally come in a variety of shapes and sizes much like our own cooking pots. Steam pots are used a lot for medicinal foods. The ingredients are put into the pot and both lids are put on and fastened by a string which passes through the handles and the pot is placed in a larger pot of boiling water. The herbs and other ingredients are cooked by the rising steam without losing any valuable elements which might be boiled out otherwise.

— Consulting a herbal practitioner —

When you make a first appointment with a Chinese herbal practitioner you may well be asked to bring with you any medical records you have and anything that could be relevant to your complaint. This does mean that the person who has the complaint has to attend. You may think this obvious but herbalists say they are constantly surprised by people who turn up and give all the symptoms and when they are asked how long they have had the complaint the herbalist will be told: 'Oh, it's not for me, it's for my aunt/uncle/brother/cousin.' So, rule 1: whoever has the complaint goes to the clinic. Unless, of course, they are too ill, in which case the herbalist may make a house call just like a doctor.

Inside the clinic

When you go in you will be greeted by what looks like an old-fashioned Western chemist's – glass display cases containing a bewildering assortment of potions, lotions, pills and packets. These are the imported Chinese generic herbs that are bought, over the counter, as remedies for coughs and colds, menstrual problems, headaches, upset stomachs, etc. – exactly the same as a packet of aspirin or a bottle of antiseptic mouthwash that you would find in your local chemist's. The difference is that the Chinese herbalist's packet of aspirin would contain the herbal equivalent and be packaged more colourfully with Chinese-style decoration and writing. A popular brand carries the Tiger logo. This can sometimes cause a herbalist a problem for when they import any of these products they are often held up at Customs in case they contain any parts of a real tiger. They don't but because the ingredients are listed in Chinese they sometimes have to be sent for analysis as tigers are a protected species.

So who buys these pre-packaged herbal remedies? Mostly Chinese customers who use them in much the same way as you would use a Western chemist's products. Each glass cabinet has a range of remedies for a particular complaint – one will have menstrual and pregnancy remedies, another children's, while another might contain remedies for male potency problems (there is even a Chinese product for over-potency).

Chinese customers will usually know what they want, and if they don't they can read the information on the packages. Westerners can't often do that so they will have to ask. Don't be in any way nervous of this. Your herbalist will be only too happy to help. They will give advice and take time to make sure you have what you need.

Beyond the cabinets of pre-packaged remedies there are the loose herbs. These are contained in large jars or in the traditional herbalist's wooden drawers. The herbs in the glass jars are obviously easy to see while the ones in the wooden drawers are hidden. None of the drawers is marked as the herbalist knows exactly what is in each one – they have to. Some of the ones in the jars may look a little strange, that's because some of them are not herbs as one would expect to see but rather dried remedies of a different kind. For example you may see dried sea-horse (very good for hangovers) or various forms of dried fish.

The loose herbs are divided into three categories:

☻ herbs for healthy eating such as adding to soups
☻ loose herbs bought over the counter instead of the pre-packaged ones
☻ herbs only supplied on prescription and usually in combinations.

The herbalist as a chemist

In the West the Chinese herbalist will do both diagnostic and prescriptive work whereas in China the herbalist will concentrate more on filling our prescriptions from doctors. Some of these doctors are herbalists themselves and others are conventionally trained doctors similar to Western ones.

The Chinese herbalist is not just a chemist though; just filling out prescriptions. They play a much more active part in the process; changing the prescription if the herbs prescribed are not in season, asking if the symptoms have changed and making adjustments accordingly, taking an interest in the general health and well-being of their clients, giving advice and information.

In the West very few GPs prescribe herbal remedies. That situation is bound to change rapidly in the near future. As more and more people come to hear and learn about Chinese herbal medicine GPs themselves will begin to show an interest in much the same way that they have with acupuncture.

Your first appointment

If it's the first time you have visited a Chinese herbal clinic you will not know which remedy it is that you need. Even if you think you do know it is best to book an appointment and have a consultation. Herbalists say a lot of their customers, especially Chinese ones, come with an idea of what they want based on what their next-door neighbour's uncle once told them might 'do the trick'. Even if your next door neighbour's uncle is a trained and qualified herbalist it is still best left to the herbalist who is actually dealing with your complaint.

When you arrive for your appointment it is unlikely that you will have to wait. You may be asked to take a seat for a moment. The herbalist, if it's your first time, will have allowed at least an hour for your consultation, if not more. If it is a subsequent visit you will be allocated less time as the herbalist already has the essential information about you and your medical history.

Herbalists usually allow at least 20 minutes between clients. This avoids keeping the next person waiting should one client over-run, or if the herbalist needs a short break. They don't usually see more than about eight people in one day – after all it is a very intensive consultation and quite exhausting at times.

The consulting room

You will be shown into the consulting room. This has to be licensed by the local authority if it is also used for acupuncture. The licence covers such aspects as hygiene, hand-washing facilities and needle sterilisation. You should check that a current local authority licence is on display.

There will probably be a couch for acupuncture and a desk with a chair for you. On the walls may well be acupuncture charts showing the meridians and acupuncture points of the human body.

Questions asked

Once the herbalist has put you at your ease, found out your name, age, etc., they will want to know about your symptoms and your complaint. They will need to know a lot of information about you – your childhood, times of the day and year you like best, foods you prefer, past medical history – that sort of thing. The herbalist needs all this information because they are not treating the complaint – they are treating you.

It is important to give the fullest possible past medical history. Don't hold anything back even if you think it is not relevant – it may well be of vital importance. Herbalists are beginning to get a lot more referrals from GPs and they are being supplied with a detailed medical history of the patient so they can work in conjunction with the GP to effect the fullest possible treatment. In the last few years the number of referrals has increased dramatically as has the number of Western clients they see. In the UK three years ago herbalists saw very few Westerners but now over 70 per cent of their clients are non-Chinese.

Examination

The Chinese herbalist may well examine you if you have physical symptoms. It's the same as a visit to the doctor. But whether you are examined or not you will certainly be closely observed. You might not even notice the herbalist doing this but they will be looking for skin colour, general body attitude, tongue colour and fur, quality and sound of your voice, emotional attitude, smell, the way you answer questions and what you wear.

You may well have your 'pulses' taken. Chinese medical practitioners feel for at least three pulses in each wrist, not just one for heartbeat as we do in the West. They will feel for the strength and regularity of each of these six pulses and can gain a lot of information about how the energy flows within us and make corrections accordingly. After treatment your pulses will be taken again to verify that change has been effected. All this information will be used to determine what type of person you are according to the Five Elements and the Harmony of the Five Sentiments. Remember it is not your complaint that is being treated but you, the whole you and nothing but you. Your herbalist will end up knowing as much about you as you do yourself – if not more.

The diagnosis

Armed with all this information the herbalist can then make a diagnosis. This is not according to Western medicine but in the Chinese way, which means your complaint will be identified as hot or cold, rising or falling, wet or dry. Chinese medical practitioners do not see a disease or a complaint in the way we do – something we catch or can't avoid, but rather as the human body being out of balance. The symptoms are just that – symptoms of a human system that is not working properly. Using herbs, acupuncture, even massage, they will restore the imbalance and return the person to full health. They will also give advice about diet, lifestyle and environment, to try and make sure that the imbalance doesn't occur again. Your herbalist will be as interested in why you have particular symptoms as they will be in the symptoms themselves.

———————— The remedies ————————

Once a diagnosis has been made your herbalist can decide what remedy will benefit you. Again it is you that is the important factor. The remedy is to restore your imbalance. It is not to kill or eradicate your complaint. Your Chinese herbalist will not see your complaint as something foreign to you, some alien force that is poisoning you, but rather as a part of you that isn't functioning as well as it might. It is to be helped back to full health rather than destroyed. There is no point waging war on yourself. You and whatever is wrong with you have to work in harmony, with your herbalist's help, to become in balance again. It is a very different approach from the one we are used to in the West where most medicine is concerned with wiping out a particular disease. Western medicine also tends to see all disease as the same: you have the flu, I have the flu; well here's the remedy for the flu – take it and it will go away. Chinese herbalists don't work that way. They would see that you and I, although both having the flu, would need different remedies as we are different people. You, and your flu, are very different from me and my flu. The Chinese see each person and their particular complaints as unique and special.

When the herbalist has made the diagnosis and selected the remedy they will give you a prescription. This will be filled out in the herbalist shop and you pay for it in the normal way. You may well be given a repeat prescription that you bring back at a later date to obtain further stocks or it may be that your herbalist will want to see you again after a week or so to see what improvement there has been. They may decide to change your remedy accordingly.

The herbalist will take into account certain factors when prescribing a treatment. They will include:

☙ Environmental factors known as the Liu Yin, the six Pernicious Influences.
☙ Special attention and care in the treatment of pregnant women since some herbs can induce premature labour or even miscarriage and some have the slight possibility of causing damage to the foetus.
☙ Any medicines prescribed may also come with advice on diet. You should adhere to this advice strictly as the herbalist may know of certain foods or beverages that could react badly with the herbal combination prescribed. There may also be advice on lifestyle which should also be considered.

From this mass of information the herbalist can make a diagnosis and issue a prescription. They will monitor the herbs used, and their effect, for as long as the remedy remains applicable to the illness.

Quantities prescribed

As with remedies being prescribed according to the patient's individual needs so the quantities prescribed will also vary from patient to patient. The quantities vary according to several factors including the patient's age, overall health, condition and whether their complaint is improving or declining. The quantities will vary from prescription to prescription because of the herbs themselves: factors taken into account will be the freshness or otherwise of the herbs, their quality generally and their combination. There are nine guidelines for prescription quantities:

1 *Health*. A normally active healthy person would expect to receive a higher dosage than a thin or frail person who has been ill for some time.

2 *Age*. Elderly patients and children would expect to receive smaller dosages than adults.

3 *Condition*. Mild cases of an illness obviously need smaller dosages than a chronic or serious case.

4 *Taste*. Strongly tasting medicines are prescribed in smaller dosages than those with little or no taste.

5 *Combination*. The main ingredient in a prescription should be in a larger dosage than the others.

6 *Category*. Ingredients derived from flowers, leaves or stems will be prescribed in smaller amounts than those from minerals, which are much denser.

7 *Method*. Boiled herbs are prescribed in much larger quantities than those supplied in pill, tablet or powder form.

8 *Season*. The dosage of the same herbs will vary according to the season that they were harvested, prepared or dispensed in.

9 *Environmental*. Where the patient lives and/or works may also affect the dosage.

Prescriptions for medicinal soups

Sometimes the herbal practitioner will prescribe a medicinal soup to be prepared at home. The ingredients will be supplied by the herbalist but the cooking conditions are not under their control. During the boiling process there is a chemical reaction between the herbs and care must be taken to follow the directions regarding boiling and simmering carefully as well as instructions regarding the order in which they are put into the pot. These procedures will be fully explained to the patient and they must be followed meticulously.

Any directions given with regard to not drinking tea while a particular course of herbs or soups is being administered should be followed carefully: tea is regarded by the Chinese as a herb in its own right and should not be combined with others if the advice is not to do so. The medicinal effects of tea, especially China teas of which there are a great variety, include removing nicotine from the body, having a diuretic effect, lowering blood sugar and assisting weight loss.

Other treatments

Your herbalist may decide that it is not a herbal remedy that you need but rather acupuncture or massage. They may be practitioners themselves or can refer you to a competent, qualified one.

Chinese medicine does not tend to have the same need for specialisation that we do in the West. Your Chinese herbalist is just as likely to be trained in acupuncture, massage and Ch'i Kung as not. They see that they have to use whatever method is necessary to help the person. Again it's a different attitude and one that takes some getting used to at first. We, the clients or patients, are the important ones and they, the practitioners, alter their approach according to our needs. If they need to refer you to an acupuncturist as they themselves don't practise then they will without a moment's hesitation if that's the best treatment for you. They won't try and prescribe herbs because that's what they sell if that's not what you need in order to effect a cure.

If your herbalist is also an acupuncturist then you will probably have your treatment in the same room as your consultation. On the first session you may have no needles at all. This is so the practitioner can spend some time assimilating all the information you have given them. They may prefer you to come back after a few days when they will have decided which acupuncture points to use.

You may have moxibustion. This is the burning, or smouldering, herb (*Artemisia japonica*) which is used to stimulate an acupuncture point instead of a needle. It's a bit like having an incense stick held quite close to your skin. It doesn't burn – it just feels warm and relieving.

If you have needles used on you then it is an interesting experience – and one that varies from person to person. The needles vary in length and the number of them used, as well as where they are used. Does it hurt? Well, again each person has a different experience. Most people say that they experience acupuncture as a relieving sort of feeling. Yes, sometimes they say it hurts but only slightly and then it's a good pain, a sort of tiny sharp pain that lasts for a fraction of a second followed by intense relief as the patient feels the meridian open and the energy begin to flow properly.

Some patients express surprise that they may attend their first appointment with their acupuncturist and not have any treatment at all. They can sometimes leave almost feeling disappointed because they didn't have any needles inserted into them. The reason for this is that sometimes the acupuncturist likes to take some time to consider their complaint, to weigh up their symptoms before deciding on a course of treatment. Sometimes they may even want to consult with a more experienced acupuncturist or one who is more familiar with dealing with a particular type of complaint. It is very different from Western diagnostic techniques where a patient may get a matter of only six minutes for a consultation with a GP and will invariably leave the surgery or clinic clutching a prescription. In the West we are only too ready to expect an instant 'cure'. A Chinese practitioner will take a lot longer to reach any conclusions or diagnosis and will take time to consider all the information before deciding on the treatment. They may even allow some time before implementing the treatment to see if the complaint responds to a climate change, a dietary change or some other external factor. They may want to see if the complaint is improving or worsening before commencing the treatment.

Properties of commonly used Chinese herbs

The Chinese name has been used along with the Western name where possible. Some Chinese herbs used are not native to the West and there is no corresponding Western name available. Where possible the Latin name has also been included. Most of the specific herbs given in this chapter can be used in their fresh state.

Tian Men Dong, *Asparagus cochinchinensis* (Asparagus)

Part used: root.
Meridians: lungs, kidneys.
Taste: bitter-sweet.
Preparation: used raw and sliced.
Purpose: to restore deficient yin. Dispels heat and strengthens the kidneys and lungs.
Usage: To treat a dry cough with little mucus, or coughing up of blood, use it with Mai Men Dong (*Ophiopogon japonicus*) and Bei Mu (*Fritillaria verticillata*) [fritillary bulb]. For use in the treatment of whooping cough with Mai Men Dong (*Ophiopogon japonicus*) and Bai Bu (*Stemona sessilifolia*) [stemona root].
Dosage: 6–12 g.

Tu Si Zi, *Cuscuta chinensis*

Part used: seeds, boiled and crushed, sometimes in cake form.
Meridians: kidneys, lungs.
Taste: sweet.
Usage: To treat deficient yang in the kidneys which causes frequent urination. Also used to prevent miscarriages and helps restore the function of the kidneys and menstrual cycle.
Dosage: 6–12 g.

Gui Zhi, *Cinnamomum cassia* (Cinnamon)

Part used: bark.
Meridian: heart, lungs, bladder.
Usage: Used in combination with Ma Huang (*Ephedra sinica*) if the patient does not sweat; if they do then give with peeled peony. Used in combination with Qiang Huo (*Notopterygium incisum*) to relieve pain in joints, especially arthritis. Use with Dang Gui (*Angelica sinensis*) [Chinese angelica] or Chuan Xiong (*Ligustrum wallichii*) to treat period pains and menstrual irregularity.
Dosage: 3–9 g (slightly more if used for arthritis).
Note: avoid during pregnancy.

Yin Yang Huo, *Epimedium brevicornu*, *E. koreanum*, *E. sagittatum*, (Barrenwort)

Part used: whole plant apart from the root.
Meridians: liver, kidneys.
Taste: sweet.
Usage: used to treat high blood-pressure in elderly women, impotency and paralysis of the lower limbs.
Dosage: 3–9 g.

Shi Chang Pu, *Acorus gramineus*

Part used: root.
Meridians: heart, spleen, stomach.
Taste: tangy.
Usage: For excess tan (mucus). Use with Zhi Zi (*Gardenia jasminoides*) [Cape jasmine], young bamboo leaves and extracted ginger juice for treating delirium. To treat tinnitus and amnesia give with Fu Ling (*Poria cocos*) and Yuan Zhi (*Polygala sibirica*) [milkwort]. For

loss of appetite give with Huo Xiang (*Agastache rugosus*), Huo Po (*Magnolia officinalis*) [magnolia] and tangerine peel.
Dosage: 3–9 g.

Qing Hao, *Artemesia annua*, *A. apiacea*

Part used: leaves.
Meridians: liver, gall bladder.
Taste: bitter but with a very pleasant smell.
Usage: For the treatment of burns and minor skin disorders use the fresh leaves crushed and applied externally. For the treatment of malaria use with Huang Qin (*Scutellaria baicalensis*) [skullcap], Ban Xin (fa) (*Pinellia ternata*) and arrowroot.
Dosage: 20–40 g for malaria, 6–15 g for skin application.
Note: this herb responds best to rapid, short boiling.

Bai Zhu, *Atractylis macrocephala*

Part used: root.
Meridians: spleen, stomach.
Taste: bitter-sweet.
Usage: to correct mischannelling of ch'i at the spleen and stomach. Used to treat loss of appetite, extended tight abdomen, vomiting and bowel disorders. It is safe to use during pregnancy.
Dosage: 4.5–9 g.

Shan Zhu Yu, *Cornus officinalis* (Cornelian cherry)

Part used: flesh of fruit.
Meridians: liver, kidneys.
Taste: bitter-sour.
Usage: Used in the treatment of abnormally heavy menstruation. Use with ginseng to treat heavy sweating accompanied by exhaustion.
Dosage: 4.5–9 g.

Tian Ma, *Gastrodia elata*

Part used: tuber.
Meridian: liver.
Taste: sweet.
Usage: To clear collateral channels and to relieve rheumatic pain. Give with Jin Yin (*Lonicera parasitica*) and Huai Nin Xi (*Achyranthes bidentata*). Give with Ban Xia (*Pinellia ternata*) and Bai Zhu

(*Atractylis macrocephala*) in the treatment of migraine, eye disorders and dizziness. Excellent for women suffering headaches, especially after childbirth.
Dosage: 3–9 g boiled in water, 1–1.5 g as a powder.

Gou Ch'i Zi, *Lycium barbarum*

Part used: seed.
Meridians: liver, kidneys.
Taste: sweet.
Usage: To strengthen Shen (life-force) and the kidneys and to improve eyesight use with Sheng Di Huang (*Rehmannia glutinosa*), Ju Hua (*Chrysanthemum morifolium*) [chrysanthemum] and Shan Zhu Yu (*Cornus officinalis*) [Cornelian cherry]. Use with Sheng Di Huang and Tian Men Dong (*Asparagus cochinchinensis*) [asparagus] to treat deficient liver and/or kidneys as well as tinnitus, dizziness, weakness of the knees and for the prevention of wet dreams.
Dosage: 6–12 g.

Xin Yi, *Magnolia liliflora* (Magnolia)

Part used: flower.
Meridians: none specific.
Taste: tangy.
Usage: For the treatment of rhinitis and nasosinusitis. Clears running nose and headaches.
Dosage: 1–3 g.

Gan Cao, *Glycyrrhiza glabra*, *G. uralensis*, *G. inflata* (Liquorice)

Part used: root.
Meridians: all.
Taste: sweet.
Usage: One of the most frequently used Chinese herbs. It can be used on its own to assist the spleen, dispel heat and restore ch'i. It is used to treat sore throats and to relieve food poisoning. It is most often used with other herbs to moderate their effects. It is also used to alleviate any uncomfortable side-effects which may be felt after taking other medicinal herbs.
Dosage: 1.5–9 g.

Ma Huang, *Ephedra sinica*

Part used: stalk.
Meridians: bladder, lungs.
Taste: tangy.
Usage: Use in combination with Gui Zhi (cinnamon) to aid sweating. Stir-fry in honey and apricot kernels to restore the function of the lungs and to suppress asthma, especially with coughing. Use with fresh ginger and Bui Zhu (*Atractylis macrocephala*) to reduce swelling.
Dosage: 3–9 g.
Note: Not suitable for patients who suffer from insomnia or high blood-pressure. Not to be used by patients who are already sweating.

Shu Di Huang, *Rehmannia glutinosa*

Part used: root (oven dried or fresh).
Meridians: liver, kidneys, heart.
Taste: sweet.
Usage: To relieve cold in the blood. Use with Xuan Shen (*Scrophularia ningpoensis*) [figwort] to reduce high body temperature, dry mouth and red tongue. Give with lotus leaves and Qian Cao Gen (*Rubia cordifolia*) for blood in vomit or urine. Use with Mu Dan Ch'i (*Paeonia suffruticosa*) [tree peony bark] for macula or dark spots on the skin. To treat thirst associated with diabetes use with Bi Xie Xu Duan (*Dioscorea batatas*) [Chinese yam] and Di Gu Pi (*Lycium chinensis*) [Chinese wolfberry].
Dosage: 9–30 g (double if fresh). Use treated (dried, then fried in rice wine until dark) for restoration of the blood, weakness of the knees, menstrual disorders and tinnitus.
Dosage: 9–15 g.

San Ch'i (also known as Tien Ch'i) *Gynura pinnatifida*

Part used: whole plant.
Meridians: kidneys, liver.
Taste: bitter.
Usage: to disperse bruises, relieving swellings and stopping hae-morrhaging, and general pain relief.
Dosage: For wounds and pain 1–1.5 g powder three times a day. For cardiac arrest 1.5 g twice a day in equal proportions with ginseng, to which this herb is similar.

Huang Ch'i, *Astragulus membranaceus* (Milk vetch)

Part used: root.
Meridians: lungs, spleen.
Taste: sweet.
Preparation: use sliced, either raw or stir-fried in honey.
Usage: To be given as a tonic to patients recovering from illness or those feeling tired and weak. Can be used in conjunction with ginseng. This is one of the most commonly prescribed herbs in Chinese medicine and symptoms which would point to its use include loss of appetite, coldness, shortness of breath and a tendency to sweat a lot.
Dosage: 9–30 g.

Yuan Zhi, *Polygala sibirica* (Milkwort)

Part used: root (chopped and treated with liquorice).
Meridians: lungs, heart, kidneys.
Taste: bitter.
Usage: for treatment of irritability, insomnia and depression.
Dosage: 3–9 g.

Zi Su Ye, *Perilla frutescens*

Part used: leaves.
Meridians: spleen, lungs.
Taste: sweet.
Usage: to promote ch'i. To relieve pain and tightness in the abdomen. To cancel out the effects of food poisoning especially caused by seafood. To ease vomiting and diarrhoea.
Dosage: 6–12 g.

Mai Men Dong, *Ophiopogon japonicus*

Part used: root nodules.
Meridians: stomach, lungs, heart.
Taste: bitter.
Preparation: used raw and pressed flat.
Usage: To restore Yin. Use with Ban Xia (*Pinellia ternata*) and liquorice for coughs and dry throat. Use with Sheng Di Huang (*Rehmannia glutinosa*), Xuan Shen (*Scrophularia nodosa*) [figwort], Huang Lian (*Coptis chinensis*) [golden thread] and Dan Shen (*Salvia multiorrhiza*) for insomnia.
Dosage: 6–12 g.

Bai Shao/ Ch'i Shao, *Paeonia lactiflora*, *P. obovata*, *P. veitchii* (Peony)

Part used: root.
Meridian: liver.
Taste: sweet.
Preparation: chopped into slices.
Usage: for abdominal pains after childbirth combine with Duang Gui (*Angelica sinensis*) [Chinese angelica], Chuan Xiong (*Ligustrum wallichii*) and Hong Hua (*Carthamus tinctorius*) [safflower].
Dosage: 6–15 g.
Note: Do not use with black false hellebore.

Yu Xing Cao, *Houttuynia cordata*

Part used: whole herb.
Meridians: kidneys, lungs.
Taste: sweet with fishy odour, also known as the fishes' smell plant.
Usage: the treatment of lung and kidney disorders.
Dosage: 9–30 g.

Mu Dan Pi, *Paeonia suffruticosa* (Tree Peony)

Part used: bark.
Meridians: kidneys, liver, heart.
Taste: bitter.
Usage: To lower high blood-pressure use with Ju Hua (*Chrysanthemum moriflorium*) [chrysanthemum] and Jin Yin Hua (*Lonicera japonica*) [honeysuckle stem]. For menstrual disorders use with Chai Hu (*Bupleurum chinensis*) and Dang Gui (*Angelica sinensis*) [Chinese angelica]. To stop bleeding in internal wounds dry fry until dark and give with Hong Hua (*Carthamus tinctorius*) [safflower]. For period pain use raw slices with cinnamon and walnuts. To stimulate the production of blood and to disperse bruises, use fired in rice wine with walnuts and cinnamon.
Dosage: 6–12 g.
Note: Not suitable for use during pregnancy.

Huang Qin, *Scutellaria baicalensis* (Skullcap)

Part used: root.
Meridians: gall bladder, small intestine, lungs, large intestine, spleen.
Taste: bitter.

Preparation: use raw or stir-fried in rice wine.

Usage: For throat pain use with Lian Qiao (*Forsythia suspensa*) [forsythia] and Jin Yin Hua (*Lonicera japonica*) [honeysuckle]. For relieving high blood-pressure use with Ju Hua (*Chrysanthemum moriflorium*) [chrysanthemum] and Nauclea rhynchophylla.

Dosage: 3–10 g.

Wu Wei Zi, *Schizandra chinensis* (northern variety), S. *sphenanthera* (southern variety)

Chinese name means 'the fruit which has five tastes'.

Part used: fruit.

Meridians: kidneys, heart, lungs.

Taste: sour.

Preparation: use raw or steamed with vinegar or rice wine.

Usage: For coughs caused by weakness of the lungs, sometimes in combination with ginseng. Use with Mai Men Dong (*Ophiopogon japonicus*) to treat patients who sweat, have a dry mouth, tire easily and are depressed.

Dosage: 1.5–6 g.

Jing Jie, *Schizonepeta tenufolia*

Part used: seeds.

Meridians: none specific.

Taste: tangy.

Usage: To stop swellings and as an excellent painkiller. Used more than any other herb for the treatment of arthritis. Fried until very dark in colour it is used to stop bleeding, especially from haemorrhoids.

Dosage: 3–9 g.

Gou Teng, *Nauclea rhynchophylla* (Gambir vine) (also Uncaria macrophylla, U. sessilifructus)

Part used: stem and thorn.

Meridians: heart, liver.

Taste: sweet.

Usage: To stop convulsions, tics and spasms use with Tian Ma (*Gastrodia elata*). For the treatment of red eyes caused by headaches use with Ju Hua (*Chrysanthemum moriflorium*) [Chrysanthemum], Sang Ye (*Morus alba*) [Mulberry leaves] and menthol. It does not need boiling.

Dosage: 6–12 g.

5

ACUPUNCTURE

*We should blunt our sharp points, and unravel the complications
of things; we should temper our brightness, and bring ourselves
into agreement with the obscurity of others. How pure and still
the Tao is, as if it would ever so continue!*

Tao Ti Ching

— Acupuncture and the meridians —

Within the body there is the balance of yin and yang and there is the
flow of ch'i. Ch'i is said to flow along lines known as meridians. Most
Chinese medicine works by accepting that the meridians conduct ch'i,
and the lines are used by acupuncturists and can be seen illustrated
in acupuncture charts.

The main difference between acupuncture and herbal medicine is that
acupuncture is concerned with stimulating and improving the flow of
energy along the meridians whereas herbal medicine is more concerned with balancing the yin and yang of the major body organs.
Acupuncture and herbal medicine are often used alongside each
other. This is because stimulating the meridian energy flow must
often be combined with balancing the yin and yang of the major body
organs. An acupuncturist may well give herbal preparations as
painkillers and a doctor may well use acupuncture to supplement
their own treatment.

In acupuncture treatment, needles are inserted at several points
along a single meridian. Another additional needle may be inserted at

the point of greatest pain, which may or may not be along the same meridian. This point of greatest pain is known as the *Hua To* after a famous doctor of the same name.

The meridian channels

There are 12 pairs of channels. They are found on both sides of the body and correspond on left and right sides.

There are:

- three yin hand channels
- three yin foot channels
- three yang hand channels
- three yang foot channels.

These are called the 12 Jin Mai or meridians. Each relates to a specific internal organ.

The Chinese include the *Sanjiao*, the triple heater, which comprises the three body cavities in their classification as an internal organ. The upper cavity is the area around the heart and lungs and corresponds roughly to the chest; the middle is the area around the spleen and stomach; and the lower is the area around the kidneys, liver, intestine and bladder. Their respective functions are:

- upper – receiving
- middle – transporting
- lower – passing or eliminating.

The 12 meridians form a complete circulatory system around the body:

- hand/lung channel (great yin)→
- hand/large intestine (yang)→
- foot/stomach (yang)→
- foot/spleen (yin)→
- hand/heart (yin)→
- hand/small intestine (yang)→
- foot/bladder (yang)→
- foot/kidney (yin)→
- hand/pericardium (yin)→
- hand/sanjiao (yang)→
- foot/gall bladder (yang)→

☺ foot/liver (yin)→
☺ hand/lung (great yin).

Each of the meridians has collateral or accompanying channels located in other parts of the body, for example the hand/large intestine (yang) channel has collateral channels in the lungs. These collateral channels could be seen as the branches of a tree and the meridian as the trunk.

Each meridian and its collaterals is linked with particular illnesses and their treatment.

The three yin hand channels

☺ Hand/lung (great yin). Collateral channels located in the large intestine. Illnesses: lung, throat and chest complaints.
☺ Hand/heart (yin). Collateral channels in the small intestine. Illnesses: heart, stomach and chest complaints, diarrhoea, mental disorders and asthma.
☺ Hand/pericardium (yin). Collateral channels in the Sanjiao. Illnesses: chest diseases, mental disorder and apoplexy.

The three yang hand channels

☺ Hand/large intestine (yang). Collateral channels in the lungs. Illnesses: high fever, high blood-pressure, ears, nose and throat, complaints of the chest and abdomen, tooth decay.
☺ Hand/sanjiao (yang). Collateral channels in the wall of the heart. Illnesses: constipation and complaints of the ears, nose and throat.
☺ Hand/small intestine (yang). Collateral channels in the heart. Illnesses: mental disorders, high fever, complaints of the neck and shoulders, eye disorders.

The three yang foot channels

☺ Foot/stomach (yang). Collateral channels in the spleen. Illnesses: of the face, mouth, teeth and throat.
☺ Foot/gall bladder (yang). Collateral channels in the liver. Illnesses: liver and gall bladder, eyes, ears and throat.
☺ Foot/bladder (yang). Collateral channels in the kidneys. Illnesses: back of the neck, the back, top of the skull and eyes.

The three yin foot channels

- Foot/spleen (yin). Collateral channels in the stomach.
  Illnesses: stomach disorders, loss of sleep and bleeding.
- Foot/liver (yin). Collateral channels in the gall bladder.
  Illnesses: complaints of the liver and gall bladder.
- Foot/kidney (yin). Collateral channels in the bladder.
  Illnesses: mental disorders and depression.

—— Internal organs – the Zang Fu ——

The internal organs of Chinese medicine are called the Zang Fu and are not to be confused with Western medicine's similar-sounding organs. The Chinese see the Zang Fu as a complete, interdependent system of the organs, the meridians and the ch'i flowing through and between them. Even their function is seen differently.

The internal organs are divided into 12. There are six Fu:

- large intestine
- small intestine
- stomach
- bladder
- gall bladder
- sanjiao (the triple warmer or three body cavities)
- the Special Permanent Fu (which is made up of the brain, marrow, bones, veins and womb).

And there are six Zang:

- kidneys
- spleen
- heart
- lungs
- liver
- pericardium (known as the heart-protector).

The 12 Zang Fu (and the Special Permanent Fu) internal organs form a complete system and they are all seen as working together to create a healthy body but each with a separate function. The two groups, Zang and Fu, are responsible for the main tasks of the human body: preserving and storing energy (ch'i); digestion; and elimination of waste.

The six Zang collectively have the task of collecting, storing and distributing energy. The six Fu are, in general, responsible for sorting out the useful from the useless substances and for getting rid of the waste. Again, don't confuse their functions, descriptions or names with those of conventional Western medicine. The differences are probably greater than the similarities.

Abilities and functions of the six Zang

The combined function of the six Zang is the preservation of energy (ch'i). Their separate functions are:

- Lungs: ruler of ch'i, energy and air; forces clearance of passages. Preserves the skin and hair.
- Kidneys: preserver of spirit (sperm); ruler of bone and water; provider of bone marrow (includes the brain).
- Pericardium: protector of the heart; governor of sex.
- Heart: ruler of pulse and spirit.
- Liver: ruler of tendons and passages; reservoir of blood.
- Spleen: ruler of the circulatory systems, including blood, skin and muscles.

Abilities and functions of the six Fu

The combined function of the six Fu is the reception, digestion, distribution and elimination of waste. Their separate functions are:

- Stomach: receiver of food and liquids.
- Bladder: reservoir and passer of urine.
- Sanjiao: Transport of food and liquids; passing of wastes.
- Gall bladder: preservation and storage of gall juice.
- Small intestine: digestion and reception of food; separating different forms of energy usage.
- Large intestine: passing of wastes.

The Special Permanent Fu

The combined function of the special permanent Fu is the conservation of ch'i. Their separate functions are:

- Veins (pulses): circulation of blood.
- Womb: female reproductive and menstrual system.

◉ Brain mental control: commands all functions.
◉ Marrow: manufacture of bones.

The yin and yang of
the Zang Fu

Each of the six Zang internal organs is regarded as being yin and the six Fu organs as yang. The Zang are the solid organs which store and the Fu are the hollow organs which transform.

As there is always a balance of yin and yang, each of the Zang and Fu are linked with a corresponding organ of the other.

◉ Spleen (yin/Zang) and stomach (yang/Fu)
◉ Lung (yin/Zang) and large intestine (yang/Fu)
◉ Kidneys (yin/Zang) and bladder (yang/Fu)
◉ Pericardium (yin/Zang) and Sanjiao (yang/Fu)
◉ Heart (yin/Zang) and small intestine (yang/Fu)
◉ Liver (yin/Zang) and gall bladder (yang/Fu).

— The five elements of the Zang Fu —

Each of these internal organs is also governed by, or comes under the influence of, one of the five elements:

◉ Earth rules yin spleen and yang stomach;
◉ Metal rules yin lung and yang large intestine;
◉ Water rules yin kidneys and yang bladder;
◉ Wood rules yin liver and yang gall bladder;
◉ Fire rules yin heart and yang small intestine.

In addition fire is said to rule the yin pericardium and the yang sanjiao.

And each of the elements corresponds to one of the Five Phases:

◉ Earth/pensiveness/spleen/stomach
◉ Water/fear/kidneys/bladder
◉ Metal/sorrow/lungs/large intestine
◉ Wood/anger/liver/gall bladder
◉ Fire/joy/pericardium/sanjiao/heart/small intestine.

The twelve primary ch'i channels

In the body, there are six yang organs and six yin organs. Each yang organ is associated with a yin organ. Paired yin and yang organs belong to the same phase in the Five Phases. Their channels are sequential to each other in the circulation of ch'i, their functions are closely related, and disease in one usually affects the other. In Chinese medicine the channel corresponding to the yang organ is often used to treat disorders of its related yin organ. In the limbs, the yang channels are on the external side of the limbs while the yin channels are on the internal side. Generally speaking, the outsides of the limbs are more yang and are more resistant and prepared for an attack, while the internal sides are more yin, and weaker.

The organs are further subdivided in order to distinguish the different levels of the yin/yang characteristics. The yang organs are divided into Greater Yang (Taiyang), Lesser Yang (Shaoyang), and Yang Brightness (Yangming). The yin organs are divided into Greater Yin (Taiyin), Lesser Yin (Shaoyin), and Absolute Yin (Jueyin).

The spleen, liver, and heart are the organs with the most direct relationship with the blood. The spleen filters the blood (modifying the blood's structure), the liver stores the blood, and the heart moves it. Any problem associated with the blood will involve at least one of these organs.

The liver and the kidney are closely related. Their channels cross in many places. The liver stores blood; the kidney stores essence. These substances, both of which are yin, have a considerable influence on the reproductive functions.

The heart (upper burner, fire) and the kidney (lower burner, water) keep each other in check and are dependent on one another. The spirit of the heart and the essence of the kidneys co-operate in establishing and maintaining human consciousness.

The spleen's digestive function is associated with the distributive functions of the liver. Disharmony between these two results in various digestive troubles. The transporting and digestive functions of the spleen (also called the Middle Ch'i) depend upon the strength of the kidney yang.

Although the lungs govern ch'i, ch'i from the lungs must mix with essence from the kidneys before original (correct, healthy) ch'i can be produced. The lungs govern ch'i, the liver spreads ch'i, and the kidneys provide its basis.

The lung channel of hand – greater yin

The lungs (yin) and the large intestine (yang) are considered paired organs. They belong to metal in the Five Phases, the westerly direction, the season of autumn, the dry climatic condition, the colour white, the pungent taste, the rank odour, the emotion of sadness, and the sound of weeping. Their opening is the nose, and they govern skin and hair.

Since the lungs belong to metal, they are able to regulate heartburn. The heart belongs to fire. Whenever the heart has excess ch'i, deep breathing is able to lead the heart's fire to the lungs, and therefore cool the heartburn. When the weather is changing from damp, hot summer into dry and cool autumn, lungs are the first organ to sense the change. If the lungs are not able to readjust to fit the new situation smoothly, you will catch a cold. The lungs access the outside world through the nose. The lungs are responsible for taking ch'i from the air, and for the energy (ch'i) state of the body.

Breathing is considered a strategy for leading ch'i to the extremities such as skin and hair. When the breathing is regulated properly, you are able to strengthen the body's guardian ch'i and generate an expansive ch'i shield to protect the body. You are also able to raise or lower the ch'i state through the breathing. For example, when you are angry, deep breathing is able to calm the excited ch'i state.

The lungs are sensitive to emotional changes, especially when you are sad or angry. They also control that part of the liquid metabolism which distributes liquid to the skin. Because the lungs are usually the first to be attacked by exogenous diseases, they are called the Delicate Organ. These diseases can also cause what is called the Non-spreading of the Lung Ch'i. The main symptom of a problem with the lungs is coughing, which is a form of Rebellious Ch'i (since the lung ch'i normally flows downward). If coughing is also accompanied by lassitude, shortness of breath, light foamy phlegm, and weakness in the voice, it is called Deficient Lung Ch'i. However, if the cough is a dry one, with little phlegm, a parched throat and mouth, and deficient yin symptoms (such as night sweating, low-grade fever, red cheeks, etc.), the condition is referred as Deficient Lung Yin.

The large intestine channel of hand – yang brightness

The lungs (yin) and the large intestine (yang) are considered paired organs. They belong to metal in the Five Phases, the westerly direction, the season of autumn, the dry climatic condition, the colour white, the pungent taste, the rank odour, the emotion of sadness, and the sound of weeping. Their opening is the nose, and they govern skin and hair. The main function of the large intestine is the metabolism of water and the passing of water. It extracts water from the waste material received from the small intestine, sends it on to the urinary bladder, and excretes the solid material as stool. Many disorders affecting this organ are categorised as spleen and stomach patterns. Certain abdominal pains are considered manifestations of a blockage of ch'i or blood in the large intestine.

The Dan Tian in the lower abdomen is considered the residence of original ch'i. In order to keep this ch'i at its residence, this area must be strong and healthy. The ch'i circulating around the intestines must not be stagnant.

The stomach channel of foot – yang brightness

The spleen (yin) and the stomach (yang) are paired organs. They belong to earth in the Five Phases, the centre, the season of long summer (the end of summer), the climatic condition of dampness, the colour yellow, the emotion of pensiveness, the taste of sweetness, fragrant odour, and the sound of joy. Their opening is the mouth and they control the flesh and the limbs.

The yin/yang relationship between the spleen and the stomach is a particularly strong example of the relationship between organs. The stomach receives food while the spleen transports nutrients. The stomach moves things downward while the spleen moves things upward. The stomach likes dampness while the spleen likes dryness.

Though there are some patterns relating to deficiency of the stomach (many of these originate in the spleen), most stomach disorders are caused from excess. Stomach fire gives a painful, burning sensation in the stomach, unusual hunger, bleeding of the gums, constipation, and halitosis.

Once saliva has begun the process of digestion, food passes to the stomach, located in the middle Sanjiao (middle triple burner) area. The stomach breaks down the food, and then passes it on to the intestines, where the essence is absorbed and converted into ch'i, and circulated through the entire body.

The stomach is related to the emotion of pensiveness. When you are upset, the stomach will not function normally. In Ch'i Kung, regulating the mind is the first step to maintaining the stomach in a healthy condition. The type of food you eat is the second consideration. The proper amount and quality of food will help you to obtain high quality ch'i to circulate in the body.

The spleen channel of foot – greater yin

The spleen (yin) and the stomach (yang) are paired organs. They belong to earth in the Five Phases, the central direction, the season of long summer (the end of summer), the climatic condition of dampness, the colour yellow, the emotion of pensiveness, the taste of sweetness, fragrant odour, and the sound of singing. Their opening is the mouth and they control the flesh and the limbs.

The spleen is the main organ of digestion. Its function is to transport nutrients and regulate the blood (regulate means to keep it within the channels). It is responsible for the transformation of food into nourishment.

When the spleen is weak, the body will not be able to use the nourishment available in food. This will cause general lassitude, fatigue, and a pasty complexion. The upper abdomen is considered the province of the spleen. Deficient spleen ch'i is shown by a sense of malaise or fullness in that area. Because it is required that the transporting function of the spleen distribute its ch'i upward, weakness in the spleen will usually cause diarrhoea. Spleen ch'i is also regarded as the Middle Ch'i, and it is responsible for holding the viscera in place. Insufficiency of the Middle Ch'i will presage prolapsed stomach, kidneys, etc. In more serious cases, the spleen yang ch'i will be deficient, which is manifested in diarrhoea, cold limbs, and abdominal pain that can be soothed by frequent warm drinks.

If any of the above symptoms are accompanied by bleeding, especially from the digestive tract or uterus, it is called Spleen Not Controlling the Blood. Cold and Dampness Harassing the Spleen is a manifestation characterised by a pent-up feeling in the chest and a bloated sensation in the abdomen, lassitude, lack of appetite and taste, a feeling of cold in the limbs, a dark yellowish hue to the skin, some oedema and diarrhoea or watery stool. The cold and dampness prevent the spleen from performing its transforming and transporting functions. This leads to a great disturbance in water metabolism and is one of the origins of phlegm.

The ultimate aim in Chinese medicine is to regulate the ch'i flow to its original (normal) level in the five yin organs. Among them, the spleen is the last and the hardest organ to regulate. It is believed that if you are able to regulate the ch'i in the spleen to a normal and healthy level, you will have grasped the key to health and longevity.

The heart channel of hand – lesser yin

The heart and the small intestine are paired organs. The heart is considered yin, and the small intestine is considered yang, balancing this paired channel. These two organs correspond to fire in the Five Phases, the southerly direction, the summer season, the climatic condition of heat, the colour red, the emotion of happiness, the sound of laughter, the taste of bitterness, and the odour of burning. Their point of entry is the tongue, they control the blood vessels and they are reflected in the face.

Almost all of the problems and disorders of the heart are associated with weakness. The four major types of heart weakness are deficient heart ch'i, deficient heart yang, deficient heart blood, and deficient heart yin.

The main functions of the heart are associated with the spirit and the blood vessels. The heart governs the blood vessels and is responsible for moving blood through them. It also stores the spirit, and is the organ usually associated with mental processes. Therefore, some forms of emotional distress, dizziness, palpitations, shortness of breath, and lack of vitality are common symptoms of heart ailments. Deficient heart ch'i is symbolised by general lassitude, panting and shallow breathing, and frequent sweating. If the face is swollen and ashen grey or bluish-green, and the limbs are cold, it is called deficient heart yang. The symptoms of restlessness, irritability, dizziness, absent-mindedness, and insomnia are typical signs of deficient heart blood. In deficient heart yin cases, developments with a flushed feeling in the palms and face, low-grade fever, and night sweating will occur.

The symptom of heart excess arises from an excess of heart fire. This is manifested by fever, occasionally accompanied by delirium, a racking pulse, intense restlessness, insomnia or frequent nightmares, a bright red face, a red or blistered and painful tongue, and often a burning sensation during urination. The latter symptom is the result of heat being transferred from the heart to the small intestine, which interferes with the small intestine's role in metabolism and the body's management of water.

It is believed that the mind is associated with the heart, and that it is also directly related to the spirit. The term heart (Xin) is usually used to represent the emotional mind or ideas. The Middle Dan Tian at the solar plexus is considered the residence of the fire ch'i. This Fire is used to nourish the brain and the spirit (Shen) at its residence, the Upper Dan Tian or third eye. In Chinese medicine it is said that the heart is the temple of the spirit because it supplies fire ch'i and can nourish the spirit without limit.

Generally speaking, the heart is very sensitive during the summertime. The heart is a yin channel, and when the summer yang comes it can increase the heart's ch'i level and cause problems. Emotional disturbances, such as excitement from happiness, are considered harmful to the heart as well, especially during the summer.

The small intestine channel of hand – greater yang

The heart and the small intestine are paired organs. The heart is considered yin, and the small intestine is considered yang, balancing this paired channel. These two organs correspond to fire in the Five Phases, the southerly direction, the summer season, the climatic condition of heat, the colour red, the emotion of happiness, the sound of laughter, the taste of bitterness, and the odour of burning. Their point of entry is the tongue. They control the blood vessels and are reflected in the face.

The major function of the small intestine is to separate waste material from the nutritious elements in food. The nutritious elements are then distributed throughout the body and the waste is sent on to the large intestine.

The small and large intestines are located in the Lower Dan Tian. In order to store the Original Ch'i converted from Original Essence, the abdomen must be healthy and the ch'i circulation in the area of the intestines must be smooth and natural. The best way to reach this goal is through abdominal breathing exercises. One such exercise is to lead the Original Ch'i upward following the heart and small intestine ch'i channels to cool down the heart fire.

The urinary bladder channel of foot – greater yang

The kidneys (yin) and the urinary bladder (yang) are paired organs. They correspond to water in the Five Phases, the winter season, the cold climatic condition, the southerly direction, the colour black, the emotion of fear, the taste of salt, the smell of decay, and the sound of groaning. Their sensory organ is the ear. Their opening is the urethra. They control the bones, marrow, and brain, and their health is reflected in the hair of the head.

The main function of the urinary bladder is to transform fluids into urine and excrete it from the body. Its pairing partner the kidney is one of the most important organs – the kidneys are the residence of the Original Essence.

The kidney channel of foot – lesser yin

The kidneys (yin) and the urinary bladder (yang) are paired organs. They correspond to water in the Five Phases, the winter season, the cold climatic condition, the southerly direction, the colour black, the emotion of fear, the taste of salt, a rotten smell, and the sound of groaning. Their sensory organ is the ear. Their opening is the urethra. They control the bones, marrow, and brain, and their health is reflected in the hair of the head.

The kidneys store Original Essence (Yuan Jing) and are therefore responsible for growth, development, and reproductive functions. They play the primary role in water metabolism and control the body's liquids, and also hold the body's most fundamental yin and yang.

Because the kidneys are the repositories of the basal yin and yang of the body, any disorder, if sufficiently chronic, will involve the kidneys. More significantly, a disease of the kidneys will usually lead to problems in other organs. Methods of strengthening the kidneys are therefore used by both medical and Ch'i Kung practitioners to increase or maintain vitality and health. The symptoms of deficient kidney yang or yin are typical symptoms of the disorder, and will appear to a certain extent as deficient yang or yin patterns in any organ.

It is easy to understand and memorise the symptoms of deficient kidney yin if one learns the correspondences of the kidneys and remembers that yin represents the constructive, nourishing, and fluid aspects of the body. Usually, the lower back is weak and sore, there is ringing in the ears and loss of hearing acuity, the face is ashen or dark, especially under the eyes. It is common to feel dizziness and thirst, and to experience night sweats and low-grade fevers. In addition, men have little semen and tend toward premature ejaculation, while women have little or no menstruation.

Deficient kidney yang symptoms are significantly associated with loss of energy or warmth. Similar to deficient kidney yin, there is commonly ringing in the ears, dizziness, and soreness in the lower back. However, the soreness is characterised by a feeling of coldness, lassitude, and fatigue. Weakness in the legs can be noticed. In men, there is a tendency toward impotence, and in both sexes, clear and voluminous urine or incontinence.

Usually, deficient kidney yin generates similar disorders in the heart and liver, while deficient kidney yang disturbs the functions of the spleen and lungs. The progression could be in the opposite direction. When this pattern is associated with the lungs, it is called 'Kidney Not Receiving Ch'i', a type of wheezing characterised by difficult breathing, mainly during inhalation. In addition to the deficient kidney yang symptoms, this condition is also manifested by a faint voice, coughing, puffiness in the face, and spontaneous sweating.

The kidneys perform an important role in the metabolism of water. If these functions are disrupted, the condition of deficient kidneys will lead to Spreading Water.

In Chinese medicine, essence (Jing) is considered the most original source of human vitality. Ch'i is converted from essence, and this ch'i supplies the entire body and nourishes the brain and spirit. It is believed that the kidneys are the residence of Original Essence. In order to protect the inherent essence the kidneys must be strengthened. Only when the kidneys are strong will they be able to keep the essence at its residence.

Maintaining the kidneys in a healthy state includes protecting the physical kidneys from degeneration, and maintaining a smooth and correct level of ch'i flow. In order to reach this goal, the diet must be considered. For example, too much salt is harmful to the kidneys, and eating too much aubergine will weaken the kidneys. In addition, the condition of the body is also important. Such things as overworking without proper rest will increase tension on the kidneys and make the ch'i flow stagnant. In winter, the kidneys will have more tension than in summer. Owing to this, the ch'i flow is more stagnant in winter than in summer. Consequently, back pain problems increase in winter.

In order to protect the kidneys, Chinese medicine practitioners have studied the relationship of the kidneys to nature, food, and even to emotional states. They have developed massage techniques and specific exercises to increase ch'i circulation in the kidneys during the winter. Since the health of the kidneys is related to the emotions as well, learning how to regulate the mind in order to regulate the ch'i is important.

The pericardium channel of hand – absolute yin

The pericardium (yin) and the triple burner (yang) are paired organs. They are said to correspond to the 'Ministerial Fire,' as opposed to the 'Sovereign Fire' of the heart and small intestine. Though the pericardium has no separate physiological functions, it is generally mentioned with regard to the delirium induced by high fevers.

The regulation of ch'i in the pericardium is considered a very important subject in Chinese medicine. It is believed that the heart, the most vital organ in the body, must have a proper level of ch'i circulation in order to function normally. The ch'i level of the heart can be raised easily to an abnormal state by illness, emotional disturbance, exercise, or injury. The function of the pericardium is to dissipate the excess ch'i from the heart and direct it to the Lao gong cavity, located in the centre of the palm. From Lao gong, the excess ch'i will be released naturally and hence, regulate the heart's ch'i level. The Lao gong cavity is used in massage to reduce the body's temperature during a fever. You can see that the purpose of the pericardium is to regulate the ch'i in the heart through the Lao gong cavity.

It should be understood that in Chinese medicine it is believed that there are five centres (called gates) where the ch'i of the body is able to communicate with the surrounding environment and, consequently, regulate the ch'i level in the body. Two of these five centres are the

Lao gong cavities, and two others are the Yong quan cavities (K-1), used to regulate the ch'i in the kidneys. The fifth one is the face. The face is connected and related to many of the organs. Whenever any of the organ ch'i is abnormal, it shows on the face.

The triple burner channel of hand – lesser yang

At least as far back as the third century AD, in the 'Classic of Difficulties' (*Nan Jing*) the triple burner was regarded as 'having a name but no form.' In the 'Inner Classic' (*Nei Jing*), it was considered to be an organ that co-ordinated all the functions of water metabolism. In other traditional documents, the burners were seen as three regions of the body used to group the organs. The upper burner includes the chest, neck, and head as well as the functions of the heart and lungs. The middle burner is the region between the chest and the navel, and includes the functions of the stomach, liver and spleen. The lower burner spans the lower abdomen, and the functions of the kidneys and urinary bladder. Therefore the upper burner has been compared to a mist which spreads the blood and ch'i, the middle burner is like a foam which churns up food in the process of digestion, and the lower burner resembles a swamp where all the impure substances are excreted.

Regulating the ch'i to a normally 'smooth-flow' state is one of the main methods for maintaining health. It is believed that the ch'i must flow around internal organs smoothly in order for them to maintain their normal functions. This means that in order to keep ch'i flow smooth and the organs healthy, you must first learn how to regulate and relax muscles that are holding and related to a given organ. External movements also exercise internal muscles. One of the most common external exercises is regulating the triple burner by lifting the hands up above the head and then moving them down slowly. These up and down arm movements extend and relax the internal muscles and thereby increase ch'i flow.

The gall bladder channel of foot – lesser yang

The liver (yin) and the gall bladder (yang) are paired organs. They correspond to wood in the Five Phases, the direction east, the spring season, the climatic wind, the colour green, the emotion of anger, the taste of sourness, the goatish odour, and the sound of shouting. Their point of entry is the eyes. They control the sinews (muscles and joints), and their health is reflected in the finger and toe nails.

The main function of the gall bladder is storing and excreting the bile produced by the liver. Together with the heart, the gall bladder is responsible for decision-making.

The main disease related to the gall bladder is a disorder affecting the flow of bile, usually caused by dampness and heat. This is commonly manifested by pain in the region of the liver, an oppressive sensation of fullness in the abdomen, and yellowish eyes, skin, urine, and tongue.

The liver channel of foot – absolute yin

The liver (yin) and the gall bladder (yang) are considered paired organs. They correspond to wood in the Five Phases, the direction east, the spring season, the climatic condition of wind, the colour green, the emotion of anger, the taste of sourness, the goatish odour, and the sound of shouting. Their point of entry is the eyes. They control the sinews (muscles and joints), and their health is reflected in the finger and toe nails.

The main task of the liver is spreading and regulating ch'i throughout the entire body. Its unique character is flowing and free. Therefore, depression or frustration can disturb the functioning of the liver. In addition, the liver is also responsible for storing blood when the body is at rest. This characteristic, together with its control over the lower abdomen, makes it the most critical organ in regards to women's menstrual cycle and sexuality.

Depression or long-term frustration can stagnate the liver's spreading function and result in continuing depression, a bad temper, and a painful, swollen feeling in the chest and sides. If this condition worsens, it may cause disharmony between the liver and the stomach and/or spleen. This disorder is symbolised by the 'rebellion' of ch'i in the latter organs, whereby ch'i moves in the opposite direction to normal. For example, the stomach ch'i normally descends, so rebellious ch'i means hiccoughing, vomiting, etc. In the case of the spleen, the ch'i ordinarily moves upward, so rebellious ch'i in this organ means diarrhoea.

Depression of the liver ch'i is the main cause of many women's disorders, including menstrual irregularities, swollen and painful breasts, etc.

One of the most important responsibilities of the liver is the storage of blood with intended emphasis upon nourishing and moistening. Whenever the liver blood is deficient, the liver will not be able to handle the function of moistening. This is generally shown as dry and painful eyes with blurred or weak vision, lack of suppleness or pain in moving the joints, dry skin, dizziness, and infrequent or spotty menstruation. If the deficient liver yin has become serious, the conditions Rising Liver Fire or Hyper Liver Yang Ascending occur. These occurrences are evidenced in ill temper, restlessness, headache, vertigo, red face and eyes, and a parched mouth. If the liver yin is so deficient that it is incapable of securing the liver yang, many of the symptoms appear as disorders of the head. Weakness in the lower joints may also be manifested.

The liver is one of the five yin organs whose ch'i level the Chinese medicine practitioner wants to regulate. Since the liver and the gall bladder are directly connected, when the liver's ch'i is regulated, the ch'i circulating in the gall bladder will also be regulated. Many methods have been developed for regulating the liver ch'i. When the arms are moved up and down, the internal muscles surrounding the liver will be moved and the ch'i around the liver will be circulated smoothly. It is believed that the liver is closely related to the mind. It is also believed that when the mind is regulated, the ch'i circulation in the liver will be normal and therefore the liver will function properly.

Diagnosis

Liu Yin: the Six Pernicious Influences

The Six Pernicious Influences are also known as the six evils although, of course, they are not evil – just natural events that only become harmful when the body cannot adjust quickly enough or strongly enough to them. They are:

- dryness
- dampness
- heat (or fire)
- cold
- wind
- summer heat.

When the balance of yin and yang are upset then the harmful effects of the Pernicious Influence can be manifested. Ch'i protects the body from Liu Yin but when the ch'i, for whatever reason, becomes weakened then illness can develop. Fever, body aches, chills and general discomfort are the signs that Liu Yin is gaining hold.

When there is actual climatic Liu Yin then it is known as External Pernicious Influence but there is also Internal Pernicious Influence where the internal organs become weakened or malfunction. Internal Pernicious Influence illnesses are usually chronic whereas External Pernicious Influence illnesses are acute and much more sudden. There is often no fever or chill accompanying Internal Pernicious Influence illnesses.

Dryness (Zao)

Dryness Pernicious Influence is usually associated with autumn and is a yang influence. Dryness is linked to dehydration and its symptoms are dry lips, nostrils and tongue, cracked skin and dry bowel motions.

External Dryness Pernicious Influence can be revealed by a dry cough with little phlegm, asthma and chest pain or a tightness of the chest as it often interferes with the descending and circulating functions of the lungs.

Dampness (Shi)

Dampness is associated with the 'long summer' which is usually damp and is a yin influence as it is heavy, slow and wet. It is associated with any damp weather or any damp conditions. Its symptoms are loss of appetite, indigestion, nausea, diarrhoea with heavy sticky bowel motions, cloudy urine, a feeling of heaviness, a 'thick' head, heavy and sore limbs, oozing skin eruptions.

External dampness will come on suddenly whereas internal dampness is much slower. They are both difficult to shift and can last a long time. They are both lingering, stagnating influences. The spleen is most sensitive to dampness, which is why most of the symptoms affect the digestive process.

Mucus (Tan) is seen as a form of internal dampness; mucus is regarded by the Chinese in a different way from Western medicine – it is seen as not just a fluid in the lungs but also as mucus of the heart which can cause mental instability and mucus of the meridians, which can cause numbness, even paralysis.

Heat (Re) or fire (Huo)

Heat is seen as the External Pernicious Influence and fire as the Internal. Heat is associated with the summer and is a yang influence. Its symptoms are high fever, skin inflammation, boils, carbuncles, a cough with thick yellow phlegm, dry tongue, unusual thirst, dry stools or burning sensations in the anus, small quantity urination, delirium, headache with swollen throat and soreness.

Cold (Han)

Cold is associated with winter and is a yin influence. Cold affects the meridians and can block the flow of ch'i and blood. Its symptoms are sharp cramp-like pains that respond to the application of heat, shivering, bluish tinge to the skin, slow movements, pronounced chills and chronic underactivity. Coldness manifests through the kidneys and the fluids affected by cold conditions such as mucus, urine, sweat, vomit and diarrhoea are seen as watery, cool, transparent or clear.

Wind (Feng)

Wind is a yang influence and is regarded in the body in the same way as it is outside the body. It is associated with spring and with movement, change and urgency. Its symptoms are pains that move from place to place, skin eruptions that appear and reappear in different locations, spasms and tremors, dizziness and twitching, sudden headaches, sore and itchy throat, congested nasal passages, numbness of the limbs, even convulsions and seizures. Wind Pernicious Influence manifesting as an Internal Influence affects the liver.

Summer heat (Shu)

Summer heat Pernicious Influence is always an external influence; it has no internal format. It is brought on by exposure to extreme heat which damages ch'i, causing exhaustion, sudden high fever, heavy sweating and loss of fluids. It is often associated with Dampness Pernicious Influence.

Lifestyle (Bu Nei Wai Yin)

All aspects of lifestyle will be taken into consideration by the herbal practitioner. The Chinese believe very strongly that how a person lives their life affects their health in a very visible way. The ideal is a lifestyle that is in harmony with the universe: one that has balance and harmony. This may not seem to be a medical matter but if the emotions are frayed by an unpleasant employment or stress caused by an unhappy relationship then the health of the individual is bound to be altered. Illness is often a manifestation of some negative quality of life and there may be no cure required beyond change.

Diet

The stomach receives food and is responsible for the beginning of the digestive process and since the spleen is responsible for transforming the food into blood and ch'i, it follows that any disruption or excess of food intake will affect these two organs which in turn will affect the whole body. Too much food taken at one time will not allow the stomach to 'ripen' or the spleen to 'transform'. This leads to Stagnant Food, which can cause belching, diarrhoea and a distended stomach.

Too much raw food strains the yang aspect of the spleen and generates internal cold and internal dampness causing abdominal pain and diarrhoea. Internal dampness and heat are caused by too much fatty or greasy food and too high an alcohol intake. Sweet foods taken in excess can also cause internal dampness and cold. Insufficient food affects the production of ch'i and blood, leading to weakness and deficient ch'i and blood.

Physical activity

There is a balance, as in all things, between too much and too little. With physical activity, and this includes general activities and not just exercise, there is also a time and a season. There is a yang time which includes morning, spring and early summer, youth and daytime. This is the time for active enterprises when blood and ch'i are strongest. There is a yin time which includes evening, autumn and winter, advancing years and night-time. This is the time for quieter activities. In the winter it is suggested that one should go to bed early and get up late whereas during the summer one should go to bed later and get up earlier. One should follow the natural rhythms of life and learn from nature: sleep when tired and be active when full of energy.

Excessive activity can strain the spleen's ability to manifest ch'i and blood, leading to a deficiency of these two substances. Excessive inactivity can seriously weaken ch'i and blood. If someone is sluggish and quiet it may be that they are displaying symptoms of weak ch'i or blood or it may be that they are causing the ch'i or blood to become weaker. Someone always excessively active could be showing symptoms of hyperactivity or they could be draining ch'i or blood. A practitioner will be able to isolate the cause.

— The Four Examinations (Si Jian) —

The Four Examinations are sometimes done formally, but often the practitioner uses intuition and casual observation to create a vivid profile of a patient. Every gesture, word and attribute provides clues to a person's health and well-being. Your practitioner will be doing four vital things:

- Looking: observing the patient's facial colour, general body type and language, the appearance of the tongue, mental state and expression.
- Listening: noting the patient's breathing, coughing and voice, the smell of the patient (the Chinese regard smell as one of the listening examinations).
- Asking: finding out the patient's full medical history, their lifestyle, their diet, sex life, fears and upbringing.
- Feeling: the Chinese practitioner feels for three pulses in each wrist which indicate the functioning of the major organs and for the palpation of the flow of Ch'i.

Looking

The practitioner will be looking for four types of visible sign:

1 general appearance
2 facial colour
3 the tongue
4 fluids.

We will now look at each of these in turn.

General appearance

This includes the patient's physical shape, their manner, the way they conduct themselves during the examination and their Shen (usually translated as spirit or life-force). The Chinese medicine practitioner spends a great deal of time asking questions. Your answers allow the practitioner to benefit from your knowledge of your own body. Questioning allows the practitioner to observe your emotions, voice and self-presentation. Basic questions focus on:

- ☺ reaction to heat and cold
- ☺ patterns of perspiration
- ☺ sleep patterns
- ☺ sexual functioning, sexual activity, and reproductive history
- ☺ medical history
- ☺ physical activity
- ☺ emotions
- ☺ if and when you experience headaches or dizziness
- ☺ type of pain, if any
- ☺ bowel and bladder function
- ☺ thirst, appetite, and tastes.

Your practitioner can tell a great deal about you from fairly simple observations. For example, forceful talkative people are regarded as yang whereas quiet reserved people are usually thought of as yin; quick movements show heat while slow movements show cold; bright eyes indicate strong Shen while dull cloudy eyes can show a weakened Shen.

Seeking clues to possible Pernicious Influences, the doctor looks for signs of heat or cold influences, excess or deficiency, yin or yang disharmonies. If a person has a heavy-footed walk, loud voice and sits in a sloppy, spread-out posture, that may indicate excess. If a person seems frail and weak, sits with shoulders slumped and is shy and withdrawn, that may indicate a deficiency. On the other hand, fast, jerky, impulsive movement and an outgoing personality indicate heat. If combined with a full, red face, high energy and a loud voice, then both heat and excess may be at work. Cold, as you might suspect, is associated with slow but not sloppy movements and a pale face. When coupled with a low voice, shortness of breath, or passivity, cold and deficiency may be at work.

Listening to the sound of a person's speech, breathing and cough can help identify a disharmony that results from one or more pernicious influences and patterns of disharmony. For example, if the voice is too loud and strident, that indicates excess, as does the sudden onset of a violent cough. A weak, low voice that doesn't project and a weak cough indicate deficiency. Losing your voice or hoarseness can indicate either deficiency or excess. Wheezing arises from dampness.

These clues can often help a practitioner make a diagnosis of the condition to be treated.

Facial colour

Ch'i and blood condition can often be seen in the facial colour. In normal healthy people the face should be 'shiny' and 'moist'. If someone is ill but the facial colour is still good then it often indicates that the illness is not severe because the ch'i and blood are not weakened. Weakened or deficient ch'i or blood will show in the face as paleness whereas excess internal heat will cause the face to glow red. Internal Dampness causes a yellow tint, and an excessive blackness, especially around the eyes, indicates that there may be a problem affecting the kidneys and that the illness will be chronic and resist treatment.

When you are feeling off-balance or have a specific disharmony, facial colours offer clues to the nature and the severity of the imbalance. There are several different methods of facial colour evaluation and the following evaluation of facial colours is derived from a combination of Chinese medicine and Five Phases principles which provides accurate analysis. The doctor will always examine your facial colours in a strong natural light rather than artificial light. The significance of facial colours is as follows:

- If the facial colour is shallow and scattered over a large area, the disease will clear up of its own accord quite quickly;
- If the facial colour is dark and cloudy, then the disease is *sinking* into the inner organs;
- If the facial colour is bright and fresh, then the disease is called *floating* and is on a superficial level;
- If the facial colour is moist, neither wet nor dry, the disease may not be severe and will be easy to treat;
- If the facial colour is dark, cloudy and dry, the disease may be severe and will be difficult to cure;
- If the facial colour is deep and accumulated in one spot, the disease may be a long-term one.

Five colours appear on the face:

- yellow
- white
- black
- red
- green.

Depending on a person's constitution, a healthy face may have one predominant colour, but several may be visible. To determine what colours are present in your face, it should always be examined in natural light. The doctor will look for the overall colour tone; study the skin to see what tones appear from under the surface; and look at any visible veins. For contrast, the doctor may well hold their hand up alongside your face.

The significance of the five colours is as follows:

- *Yellow* is the colour associated with the spleen system. If the face appears light yellow, then the spleen system is damp and hot. If the face appears deep yellow, heat has accumulated. If it is dark yellow, heat is the result of Xue stagnation (blood vessel collapse). Withered yellow indicates a heat deficiency.
- *White* is the colour associated with the lung system, which regulates ch'i, the breathing in of oxygen, and the exhalation of carbon dioxide. If a person is not able to exhale completely, as in emphysema, their face will take on a greyish-white colour. If the person inhales poorly, then the face will appear pale and lustreless.
- *Black* is the colour associated with the kidney system. If the face is cold and black, the kidney system is not filtering Xue properly. If the face colour is black but bright and moist, the condition can be treated. If the face is not shining, the condition is not good. If the face is withered, the kidney system yin is dry. If the face is cloudy and dark, the kidney system yang is dying.
- *Red* is the colour associated with the heart organ system and Xue. If the face is a fresh red, the Xue is hot. If the face is dark red, the Xue is stagnant. If it is light red, the Xue is deficient.
- *Green* is the colour associated with the liver system and circulation of the Xue. If veins on the face appear greenish purple, the Xue is hot. If the veins appear greenish black, the Xue is stagnant. If the condition is severe, the veins on the face appear black.

Occasionally, there are combinations of colours. This further refines the evaluation. For example, if the colour is red and white, both the heart and lung channels are involved.

The tongue

Studying the tongue is regarded as one of the most important factors in patient examination. It is regarded as the only internal organ that can be seen under normal circumstances. The tongue is seen in two parts: the tongue itself and the 'fur' that is on it. A normal tongue is pink, indicating good blood flow. The fur should be thin and moist and the tongue proper should be visible through it.

The size of the tongue will also be considered as well as its movement and general strength. Also each area of the tongue is seen as reflecting the general health of an internal organ: the tip for the lungs, the very tip for the heart, the centre for the spleen and stomach, the sides for the gall bladder and the root for the kidneys.

The tongue is the mirror of the body. Harmony and disharmony are reflected in the tongue's colour, moisture, size and coating and in the location of any abnormalities. Healthy organ systems and a lack of External Pernicious Influences produce a healthy tongue, which is pinkish red, neither dry nor too wet, fits perfectly within the mouth, moves freely and has a thin white coating. Imbalances in the organ systems and/or invasion by Pernicious Influences produce an unhealthy tongue. External Pernicious Influences produce changes in the tongue coating. Interior problems, such as organ system or Essential Substance disharmonies, produce changes in the tongue body.

When examining the tongue, the practitioner looks at the colour of the tongue body, its size and shape, the colour and thickness of its coating or fur, locations of abnormalities, and moistness or dryness of the tongue body and fur. These signs not only reveal overall states of health but correlate to specific organ functions and disharmonies, especially in the digestive system. To evaluate the tongue accurately, always do the examination in natural light.

Tongue body
The tongue body is a fleshy mass and has colour, texture, and shape independent from the apparent qualities of the tongue coating. The practitioner will look out for several indicators:

- A pale tongue body indicates deficient Xue, ch'i, or yang or excess Cold. An overly red tongue body indicates excess Heat.
- A purple tongue indicates that ch'i and/or Xue are not moving harmoniously and are stagnant.
- Pale purple means the stagnation is related to Cold. Reddish purple is related to stagnation of heat.
- When the tongue is black or grey, it indicates extreme stagnation; if black and dry, that indicates extreme heat stagnation; if black and wet, that indicates extreme cold stagnation.
- Bright red indicates deficient yin or excess heat. Dark red indicates

excess heat. Cracks in a red tongue indicate deficient yin or heat injuring the fluids. If the tongue is pale and cracked, there is deficient ch'i or Xue.

☙ Thorny eruptions of the buds on the tongue alert the doctor to heat or stagnant Xue.

Tongue fur

The tongue's coating is best described as moss or fur. It arises when the spleen causes tiny amounts of impure substances to drift upward to the tongue. When the spleen and stomach are in balance, there is a uniform density of fur, with a slightly thicker area in the centre of the tongue. Signs to look out for are as follows.

☙ A greasy fur is a sign of mucus or dampness in the body.
☙ If the fur looks peeled off or missing, it reveals deficient spleen, yin or fluids.
☙ White, moist fur indicates Cold. However, white fur resembling cottage cheese, points to Heat in the stomach.
☙ Thick fur indicates excess.
☙ Thin fur is related to deficiency during illness, but is normal if you are well.
☙ Wet indicates excess Jin-Ye (fluids) and/or a deficient yang.
☙ Dry fur is a sign of excess yang or deficient Jin-Ye.
☙ Yellow fur means heat.
☙ Grey/black fur with a red body is associated with extreme heat; grey/black fur with a pale body is a sign of extreme cold.

Shape and Size

The healthy tongue should rest comfortably in the mouth. It shouldn't be too large or too small. There are various telltale signs of disease in the tongue's shape and size:

☙ If it swells so that it fills the mouth and is deep red, that means excess heat in heart and spleen are a problem;
☙ A small, thin tongue indicates deficient yin or Xue;
☙ If a tongue is flabby and enlarged, it can indicate deficient ch'i;
☙ If, in addition to being flabby and enlarged, the tongue has scalloped (or tooth-marked) edges, then it indicates dampness due to deficient ch'i or stagnation of fluids;
☙ If the tongue is enlarged and hard, it is a sign of excess ch'i.

Movement

The way the tongue moves is also an indicator of disease.

☙ A trembling, pale tongue indicates deficient ch'i.

- A flaccid tongue that is pale often reveals extreme ch'i or Xue deficiency.
- A flaccid tongue that is deep red reveals severe yin deficiency.
- A trembling, red tongue indicates interior wind.
- If the tongue sits off-centre in the mouth, early or full-blown wind stroke may be present.
- A rigid tongue accompanies an Exterior Pernicious Influence and fever. This may indicate the invasion of the pericardium by heat and mucus obstructing the heart ch'i.

Location of abnormalities

The location of disturbances on the tongue are vivid indications of where disease is likely to be located. Certain organs are associated with the upper, middle and lower triple burner, which are in turn associated with the front, middle and back sections of the tongue. For example, if the tip of the tongue is red it indicates heat in the heart. If there are red spots on the front third of the tongue, which is associated with the upper burner, this indicates that there is heat in the lungs. Menstrual cramps, when associated with stagnant Xue, are often accompanied by purple spots on the edges of the tongue in the liver/gall bladder area.

The role of tongue diagnosis

Not all tongue irregularities are indications of disharmony, however. Food and drugs may change the coating or colour of the body of the tongue. For example, coffee yellows the coating, tobacco smoke can fur the tongue up, and some stomach anti-acidics turn the tongue black.

Furthermore, some people have minor, unchanging cracks on their tongue, which are considered normal. Others are born with what is called a geographic tongue, which is covered with severe cracks and covered with raised lumps and depressions – known as *hills and valleys*. This is considered normal by some practitioners, but a sign of congenital disharmony by others.

The way a tongue appears is not an absolute indicator of the location of the disharmony, but when taken as part of an overall pattern that includes a complete evaluation, it offers strong clues to the location of disharmony.

Fluids

These include phlegm, vomit, sweat and saliva. The practitioner will examine these if they need to. Urine and faeces are classified under

'Asking' as Chinese practitioners rarely request, or examine, specimens in the way that Western doctors do. They rely on a patient's description.

Listening

Included with listening is 'smelling'. The practitioner is listening to the tone and quality of the voice: is it strong or does it whine? Is it expressing the facts clearly and forcefully or does it stammer and sound weak? A loud, clear voice is seen as yang while a quiet voice is seen as yin. The practitioner will also be listening to see if the voice matches the patient. They will also listen to the patient's cough and their breathing.

The smell of a patient is important as it can lead to a diagnosis because it indicates the predominate element of the patient. Sometimes the doctor may even need to taste the patient to confirm a diagnosis. The five elements, smells and tastes are:

- wood/rancid/sour
- fire/scorched/bitter
- earth/fragrant/sweet
- metal/putrid/pungent
- water/rotten/salt.

Some of the names may appear rather emotive but it is just their translation. A Chinese practitioner would mentally use the Chinese equivalents and not think of someone as 'rotten' or 'rancid'.

Asking

Your practitioner will want to know about your medical history and your urine and stool quality, location and type of pain, appetite and tastes, sleep patterns, eating and drinking preferences and feelings of hot and cold. Obviously the medical history is the most important but so are the questions regarding hot and cold because they point towards identifying the Pernicious Influences and they also help characterise yin and yang qualities. For internal disorders cold generally corresponds to yin, and hot to yang. Feeling warm to the touch or a dislike of heat can point to a sign of the External Pernicious Influence of heat or summer heat, while feeling cold to the touch or a dislike of the cold can point to a sign of the External Pernicious Influence of cold or dampness.

The condition of pain is also important, especially when linked to the feelings of hot and cold. Generally pain lessened by heat signifies cold, and pain lessened by cold signifies heat. Pain with sensations of heaviness signifies dampness; pain moving around signifies wind; superficial pain with tiredness signifies dampness, as does pain which intensifies in humid weather.

Hunger and thirst are also important: thirst is a sign of heat and lack of thirst one of cold. Excessive appetite is a sign of Internal Pernicious Influence of fire while a low appetite usually signifies Dampness.

Feeling

Apart from actually feeling the patient's skin to ascertain whether they feel hot or cold the practitioner will also 'take the pulses' of the patient. This is the most important aspect of feeling. This taking of the pulses is much more involved than pulse taking in the West. The Chinese practitioner will be feeling for three pulses in each wrist. They do this with the first, index and middle finger of one hand with their thumb resting lightly across the back of the patient's hand.

The pulses are felt for three levels of pressure:

- *Deep.* Quite hard pressure, pushing hard down onto the skin;
- *Middle.* Moderate pressure, similar to a Western Doctor taking a pulse;
- *Superficial.* Light pressure, barely touching the skin.

The right wrist	1	First pulse	Lungs
	2	Second pulse	Spleen
	3	Third pulse	Kidney yang (Life Fire Gate)
The left wrist	4	First pulse	Heart
	5	Second pulse	Liver
	6	Third pulse	Kidney yin

The three pulses at three different pressures in two wrists (18 pulses) are further classified into 28 different types (504 pulse combinations) which are felt for various factors including speed, rhythms, strength, width, quality, shape and length.

With this many combinations it is a very skilled process, and one in which it takes many years of experience to become fully adept.

The 28 pulse combinations are:

1 Floating (*fu mai*) – yang pulse signifying deficient yin or interior wind;

2 Sinking (*chen mai*) – yin pulse signifying internal disharmony;

3 Swift (*shu mai*) – yang pulse signifying heat accelerating the movement of blood;

4 Slow (*ch'i mai*) – yin pulse signifying cold or insufficient ch'i;

5 Hollow (*kong mai*) – yin pulse signifying deficient blood or extreme blood loss;

6 Diffuse (*san mai*) – yin pulse signifying exhausted kidney yang;

7 Thin (*xi mai*) – yin pulse signifying deficient ch'i and/or deficient blood;

8 Large (*da mai*) – yang pulse signifying excess heat in the stomach;

9 Empty (*xu mai*) – yin pulse signifying deficient ch'i and blood;

10 Full (*shi mai*) – yang pulse signifying excess;

11 Waxy (*hua mai*) – yang with yin pulse signifying excess of dampness;

12 Choppy (*se mai*) – yin pulse signifying congealed blood;

13 Moderate (*huan mai*) – yin/yang pulse signifying normality;

14 Flooding (*hong mai*) – yin within yang pulse signifying fluids injured by heat;

15 Tiny (*wei mai*) – yin pulse signifying extreme deficient ch'i;

16 Frail (*ruo mai*) – yin pulse signifying deficient ch'i;

17 Moist (*ru mai*) – yin pulse signifying deficient blood or internal dampness;

18 Toughened (*ge mai*) – yin pulse signifying deficient blood;

19 Hidden (*fu mai*) – yin pulse signifying deficient yang or cold obstructing the meridians;

20 Confined (*lao mai*) – yang within yin pulse signifying obstruction due to cold;

21 Twisting (*dong mai*) – yang pulse signifying heart palpitations or extreme fright;

22 Wiry (*xuan mai*) – yang pulse signifying a disharmony of gall bladder and liver;

23 Tight (*jin mai*) – yang with yin pulse signifying excess cold;

24 Short (*duan mai*) – yin pulse signifying deficient ch'i;

25 Long (*chang mai*) – yang pulse signifying excess ch'i;

26 Knotted (*jie mai*) – yin pulse signifying cold obstructing ch'i;

27 Hurried (*cu mai*) – yang pulse signifying heat agitating ch'i and blood;

28 Intermittent (*dui mai*) – yin pulse signifying exhausted organs.

Diagnosis by excesses and deficiencies (Bian Zheng)

The practitioner will be looking for excesses and deficiencies in four main areas: ch'i, heat and cold, yin and yang, and blood.

- Deficient ch'i: weakness, lethargy, bright pale face, weak pulse, pale tongue, soft voice.
- Excess ch'i: localised soreness, swelling, dark or purple tongue, wiry or tight pulse.
- Deficient heat: reddish tongue, rapid thin pulse, weakness, slight fever, insomnia, dark urine.
- Excess heat: high fever, rapid or full pulse, constipation, dark and meagre urine, delirium, thick yellow fur on tongue, reddish tongue.
- Deficient cold: weakness, frailty, abundant and clear urine, thin tongue fur, puffy tongue, pulse slow and weak, weak Shen.
- Excess cold: pulse slow and strong, pale tongue, thick white tongue fur, slow movements, clear insufficient urine, cold limbs.
- Deficient yin: dizziness, impaired vision, numb limbs, thin body, thin pulse, pale face, dry skin, dry hair, limbs tremble.
- Excess yin: pulse slow and strong, pale tongue, thick white tongue fur, slow movements, clear insufficient urine, cold limbs.
- Deficient yang: weakness, frailty, abundant clear urine, thin tongue fur, puffy tongue, pulse slow and weak, weak Shen.
- Excess yang: high fever, rapid or full pulse, constipation, dark meagre urine, delirium, thick yellow fur on tongue, reddish tongue.
- Deficient blood: dizziness, impaired vision, numb limbs, thin body, thin pulse, pale face, dry skin, dry hair, limbs tremble.
- Excess blood: blood in the urine, vomit, phlegm or faeces, thirst, rapid pulse, irritability, scarlet tongue, delirium.

The symptoms for excess cold and excess yin are identical. So, too, are deficient yin and deficient blood, deficient cold and deficient yang, excess yang and excess heat. As well as the excesses and deficiencies mentioned there can also be excesses and deficiencies of all the major organs as well as the Pernicious Influences. The basic formulae is Yin = Interior/deficient/cold whereas Yang = Exterior/excess/hot; Yin = weak/pale/thin, Yang = strong/dark/thick.

There are two other classifications:

- Congealed blood: haemorrhaging, tumours and lumps, dark face, dark purple tongue with red spots, choppy pulse.

☺ Stagnant ch'i: usually resulting from emotional or dietary causes. Ch'i stuck in a particular meridian or organ. Distended swellings and soreness. Dark or purple tongue, wiry or tight pulse.

Organs and diagnosis

Liver and gall bladder

The liver controls the movement of energy throughout the body. Excess yang in the liver will result in severe headaches, red and painful eyes and hearing disorders. A disordered liver can result in blood being vomited. Blurred eyesight may be a sign of liver disease. Healthy liver blood can be seen in the fingernails: if they are red and healthy then so is the liver blood. In Chinese medicine the gall bladder and the liver are treated as one organ. A disordered gall bladder may result in bitter gall juices being vomited.

Lungs and large intestine

The lungs control the distribution of ch'i and when disordered result in asthma, shortness of breath, a low weak voice, a lack of patience, and laziness. The lungs and large intestine are seen as connected as they both provide passage. The nose is seen as the external visible sign of lung and large intestine function as well as the voice.

Heart and small intestine

The tongue and the colour of the face are seen as the external visible signs of heart and small intestine function. Impaired heart function can also be detected by loss of memory, fear, nervousness and abnormal gestures as well as by pulse condition. If the heart's energy is weakened the pulse will be weak or lacking in strength; if the energy is uneven the pulse feels irregular and lacking in rhythm.

Spleen and stomach

The lips are said to be the external visible sign of spleen function. A weakened spleen affects the appetite and causes a lack of strength in the hands and feet. It can also cause excessive thinness with the lips being white or pale yellow. Stomach disorders can produce toothache.

Kidneys and bladder

The kidneys control the bones, and the teeth are seen as the 'ends of the bones'. Kidneys are also known as 'Fire at the Gate of Life'. Hearing disorders and constipation can also result from kidney disorders.

Excess kidney function can cause sexual over-indulgence and irritability. Deficient kidney function can cause impotency, premature ejaculation and unnatural passivity. Normal kidney function can be determined from the condition of the hair, as can the bladder function.

____ Techniques of acupuncture ____ stimulation

Zhen (needle) = acupuncture; it literally means needle puncture (*acus* = needle) but the term has a more general meaning: stimulation of specific acupuncture points in the superficial areas of the body by many different methods. Jiu (fire = moxibustion) is the direct or indirect application of heat to the acupuncture points. The most important aspect of acupuncture is not the precise method of stimulation but to apply an adequate stimulus to the correct points.

Using needles (Zhen)

In traditional acupuncture, nine types of needles were used. Some of these were like scalpel blades or lances and must have been very painful indeed. These are seldom if ever used in Western acupuncture today. To avoid unnecessary suffering, the finest needles possible should be used. In practice this means using 25–32 gauge needles for children and 19–25 gauge needles for adults.

The length of the needles depends on the condition being treated and on the location of the points to be needled. Points over bony areas, such as the scalp, face, ears and distal limbs require the shortest needles. Those over the thorax, abdomen and lightly muscled areas require medium length needles and those over heavily muscled areas, such as the lumbar area, the hindquarter (buttock and thigh) area and the heavy muscles of the shoulder area require the longest needles.

In general, needle lengths ranging from 10–50 mm should suit all purposes in children and needles 10–100 mm should suit all purposes in adults. In human surgery under acupuncture analgesia, occasionally very long (up to 250 mm) needles are placed parallel to the incision site, one on each side of the wound. The needles are made of very high quality stainless steel wire. The cheapest needles are made in China and Taiwan but many other Eastern and Western countries make them. They are available through acupuncture supply houses.

Acupuncture needles are expensive and between 1 and 20 may be required during a session. If 6–12 needles are bent or destroyed each time, the cost can be high. Therefore, the thicker needles (19–25g) are used in adults. Even then, some of them will be bent during therapy. Chinese (Yuan Li) needles, 30 mm long and 21 gauge wide are ideal for use in adults.

Before use, each needle should have been properly sterilised. It should be checked to ensure that it has no physical defects such as a blunted or hooked tip, bent or rusted body or loose handle. The points are clipped and cleaned with alcohol or other antiseptic solution.

Acupuncture needles are inserted by a push-twirl technique in two stages: the first movement to penetrate the skin and the second to place the needle to the required depth in the tissues. With longer needles, it is useful to hold the needle shaft with one hand about 25 mm from the tip (using a cotton-wool bud or piece of sterile tissue) and to push-twirl the handle of the needle with the other hand. Alternatively, a stainless steel or plastic needle guide can be used. Needle guides are hollow tubes, about 10-13 mm shorter than the needle. The guide is placed firmly on the point and held with one hand. The needle is inserted into the tube and the needle-handle, protruding from the guide, is tapped firmly with the finger of the free hand to drive the needle 10-13 mm deep. The guide is then removed and the needle is advanced to the correct depth.

It is not possible to give an exact depth or direction for needle insertion: these vary between points. The direction of insertion depends on the body region being needled. Over muscular areas, the needle is usually inserted at a right angle to the skin, deep into the muscle. Over bony areas and on earpoints, the needle is inserted perpendicularly until the skin is penetrated and then is advanced subcutaneously. One should not normally needle the periosteum (except in cases where this is specifically indicated) or the ear cartilage. Accidental striking of bone can bend the tip of the needle, making it difficult to extract and destroying the tip.

Penetration of the human ear cartilage can cause a chronic auricular chondritis which can be very difficult to cure. In animals (because ear acupuncture is less commonly used than in humans) this problem is uncommon, but it is safer to avoid penetrating the cartilage. Penetration of the thoracic or abdominal cavities is normally forbidden, except in specific cases, such as aspiration of fluid or releasing gas from the viscera, etc. Therefore, when needling points over the thorax and abdomen, the needles are usually inserted at 45 degrees, to reduce the risk of accidental penetration into the cavity. Penetration of major arteries (such as the carotid) or of sensitive organs such as the eye is forbidden.

The depth of insertion also varies. In adults the needles can be inserted up to 100 mm deep in certain points, such as those over heavy muscles, or when the needle is obliquely inserted in certain points on the head. However, depths of 25-50 mm would be more usual. Certain points are merely pricked to a depth of 3 mm or so.

In children, heavy muscle groups would be needled to depths of 10–50 mm, depending on the amount of muscle. Pricking of certain points and shallow needling (up to 10 mm deep) of other points is applied.

The most active points are over peripheral nerves especially main nerves, such as the trigeminal, facial, radial, median, ulnar, sciatic, spinal nerves, etc. Nerves running on and in the muscles are also very important. The acupuncturist deliberately inserts the (very fine) needles directly through these nerves. Nerve stimulation (by twirling the needle clockwise and anticlockwise and pecking it up and down) causes very specific sensations (De ch'i), by which one knows that the correct spot has been located. Shooting sensations (paraesthesia), numbness and heaviness must be elicited, otherwise the needle is not exactly in the correct position. Once the needle is correctly in the nerve point and De ch'i has been attained, care is taken to avoid further pecking motion with the needle to avoid physical damage to the nerve. This is more important when hypodermic needles (with sharp cutting edges) are used.

When the needle is correctly placed and stimulated, a local reflex muscle spasm grips the needle tightly, 'like a fish taking the bait'. The response is felt both by the patient and the acupuncturist.

Tonification and sedation techniques

Classic methods of manipulating the needle are different if the diagnosis indicates a definite excess of ch'i in a meridian (Shi diseases = excess ch'i) or definite deficiency of ch'i in a meridian (Xu diseases = deficient ch'i). In Shi diseases use Xi (sedation) technique. In Xu diseases use Bu (tonification) technique. In both methods, the needle is manipulated until De ch'i arrives, i.e. until sensation of tingling, numbness, heaviness and gripping sensation needle occurs.

In Bu (tonification) technique the needle is thrust in heavily and rapidly. It is rotated (twirled) with small amplitude and low frequency and is lifted gently and slowly before the next rapid and heavy thrust.

In Xi (sedation) technique the needle is thrust in gently and slowly. It is then twirled strongly (large amplitude) at high frequency and is lifted forcibly and rapidly before the next gentle and slow thrust.

Duration of needling

Needles are usually left in position for 10–30 minutes in conditions such as rheumatism, muscle pain, arthritic lameness, etc. Occasionally the practitioner may be too busy to wait for up to 30 minutes until the needles are withdrawn. In these cases the patient may be instructed to twirl the needles for 10 seconds every 2–4 minutes, until 10–30 minutes have elapsed and to remove the needles then. (In this case, disposable needles are used.) In some cases, for instance rhinitis, conjunctivitis, shock, etc., duration of needling can be very short – 10–60 seconds.

In general, for paralysis and painful conditions (especially of the muscles) long duration of needling (up to 30 minutes) is indicated, whereas for most other conditions a quick needling is sufficient. Some practitioners suggest that if De ch'i is obtained, there is no advantage to be gained from leaving the needles *in situ* for 10–30 minutes, except in certain chronic conditions, such as peripheral nerve damage. Thus a short, quick, strong needling may replace the longer, more gentle method in many diseases.

Needles falling out

If a needle that has been properly inserted falls out during treatment, it is usually left out. Relaxation of the muscles around the needle is taken to indicate sufficient stimulation for that point.

Other types of needling

Traditionally two other types of needle have been used – the blood needle and the fire needle. The blood needle is a thick needle or lance used to puncture points over superficial blood vessels to allow a small amount of blood to escape. A mild haematoma around the puncture would cause longer stimulation of the point than if a fine needle were used. However this method has few adherents at best. The fire needle is a thick needle which is heated before use by burning a swab soaked in alcohol on the needle. It is then plunged in the tissues, taking special precautions. This method is seldom used in the West.

The moxa needle method is used widely, especially in muscle rheumatism and 'Cold Diseases'. In this method, standard acupuncture needles are inserted into the points as usual. A piece of moxa about 20 mm long and 20 mm diameter is pushed over the handle of the needle and is ignited. The moxa burns slowly for 5–10 minutes and the heat is transferred to the needle and the tissues. This method is not painful and does not usually cause noticeable tissue damage. At the end of the session the patient may be sweating profusely near the needle site and occasionally in other areas if multiple needles are used. (It is well known that heat applied to the trunk will cause reflex sweating of the face.)

Point injection

This has two advantages: it is much quicker to use than classic needling and electro-needling; it produces stimulation which lasts for up to an hour or more after injection.

The points are chosen in the usual manner. Standard precautions of needle sterility and skin cleanliness are taken, and sterile solutions are used. Disposable 19–25 gauge needles are inserted to the correct depth. The needles are manipulated to elicit the needle reaction (De ch'i) as described before. Then a syringe is attached and 1–10 ml of solution is injected. Small volumes are used in children and on earpoints. Larger volumes are used in adults and in muscular areas.

If orthodox drugs, suitable for intramuscular injection (such as antibiotics, hormone solutions, electrolyte solutions, etc.) or plant extracts (as in Chinese herbal medicine) are indicated, they can be diluted, as needed, before injection into the points. Alternatively they can be given subcutaneously over the points if they are suitable for subcutaneous injection. Some practitioners claim that drugs injected at the correct acupuncture points have clinical effects at much smaller dose rates than if they were injected in random (usual) sites. This claim has yet to be fully tested.

Injection of scar tissue

If the acupuncture point is in a tender area of scar tissue (especially where there is marked twisting or distortion of tissue on a major meridian), this can be quickly treated, using a dental or tuberculin syringe, set to deliver 0.1–0.2 ml/point. The solution (Impletol or Procaine solution) is injected intradermally at a depth of 2–5 mm, using a very fine (c. 25 gauge), short (2.5–10 mm) needle. The scar is injected at intervals of approximately 4 mm along its length – about 11 shots along the length of a 40 mm scar. Some experts inject straight into the centre of the scar. Others inject from the periphery towards the centre. Still others inject only the tender (sensitive) parts of the scar.

If one does not wish to inject scar tissue, one may still re-establish the flow of ch'i through the area by a technique known as 'Bridging the Scar'. The needles are left in position for up to 20 minutes and are then removed. The scar is treated 3–6 times at intervals of 2–7 days.

Implants and nerve massage

In acupuncture sterile foreign bodies are sometimes implanted in the tissues at acupuncture points to elicit long-term stimulation in chronic diseases, such as chronic bronchitis and asthma. Stainless steel acupuncture needles and other special steel implants may be used. They are anchored externally or internally so that they can be removed easily, if required. Absorbable material such as catgut and foetal or placental tissue is also used. In this method a curved suture needle is used to introduce the material in through the active point and out through another, such as Fei Shu (BL 13) and Chueh Yin Shu (BL 14) in asthma. The ends are cut off at the skin and the skin is massaged to bury the material in the tissues, where it is left until it is absorbed by the body. It could be used in chronic conditions of the lumbo-sacral and sacroiliac region and chronic gastric and pulmonary conditions.

Other types of implant include press needles, acupuncture staples and gold beads. Press needles and intradermal needles are made of stainless steel, usually 30–32 gauge. Press needles may be 1 or 2 mm long. Intradermal needles may be up to 10 mm long. They are inserted into the dermis and are taped in position for 1–6 weeks, depending on the condition being treated. Press needles are used especially on ear acupuncture points. Intradermal needles (5–10 mm long) may be used on ear or body points (but usually on the body points). They are used especially in chronic diseases and chronic pain. For instance to counteract withdrawal symptoms when cigarette smokers give up the habit, press needles may be put in ear points Lung and Shenmen and left in for 2–4 weeks. In asthma, intradermal needles may be put in points PC 06, NX 04, CV 17, BL 13, and press needles in earpoints Lung or Asthma. Intradermal needles are left in position for 1–2 days in summer and for longer periods in winter. Care must be taken to prevent local infection at the needle sites.

Incision of certain acupuncture points, leaving a 10–25 mm wound in the skin down to the subcutaneous layer, is used in certain chronic conditions. An example is Yu Ch'i (LU 10) in chronic asthma.

Incision, with exposure of the nerve and blunt massage of the nerve using artery forceps, is used in poliomyelitis paralysis in China. For instance incision of Chien Cheng (SI 09) over the junction of the radial, median and ulnar nerves above the posterior axillary crease is used in paralysis of the upper limb or difficulty in raising the shoulder. Other points which may be treated in this way in very serious cases are Ho Ku (LI 04) and Chu Chih (LI 11) near branches of the radial nerve; Huan Tiao (GB 30) near the superior gluteal nerve; Yang Ling Chuan (GB 34) near the tibial and common peroneal nerves and ST 36 near the deep peroneal nerve.

— Selection of acupuncture points —

Acupuncture treatment is administered at specific points or sites on the body. For this reason, the selection and combination of points in an acupuncture prescription is most important. At the same time the physician must be able to choose flexibly between one or more acupuncture methods, depending upon the characteristics of the disease. Following is a summary of point selection and combination strategies, together with clinical applications.

Principles of point selection

Point selection may be divided into four broad groupings:

- points chosen for particular symptoms
- specific point usage
- local points chosen in the vicinity of the disease
- distal points chosen away from the disease.

In practice, each may be used in combination with, or independent of, the others.

Local point selection

Local refers to the vicinity of the pain. Thus, pain in the head, neck forearm, low abdomen, knee, foot, etc., can be treated via points in the same locality. Diseases of the limbs and superficial diseases of the body are commonly treated by this method.

Pain of the knee can be treated at local points GB 34, Sp 9, Sp 10, St 34, Xi Yan (St 35 with other side of patella). GB 34 is the influential points of the tendons. Pain of the wrist is needled at SJ 4, SJ 5, or LI 5, SI 6. Many diseases of the head and body may also be treated through local points. Eye diseases can be treated at UB 1, GB 1, and ear diseases at SJ 21, SI 19, GB 2; asthma at Ren 22, UB 13, Stomach ache at Ren 12, St 21, UB 21.

The efficacy of needling local points to treat disease can be explained not only on the basis of traditional channel theory, but more recently by neural segment theory as well. For example in acupuncture anaesthesia, the point SI 18 is used for surgery on the cranium, and the point LI 18 for operations on the thyroid. Similarly in the clinical treatment of diseases of the viscera, it is common to select a vertebral point on the same horizontal plane as the affected organ. Choosing a point in the same or neighbouring neural segment as that of the pain or disease is also compatible with the rules of traditional local point selection.

Distal point selection

The technique of needling distal points is related to the channel theory of root and branch, whereby a disease above is treated by a point below, and vice versa. Distal refers to a location far from the site of the pain, usually a point below the elbow or knee. The method is commonly used to treat diseases of internal organs: Lung 6 for coughing blood; PC 6 for chest pain; ST 36 for abdominal pain. This method may also be used for diseases of the head and trunk.

LI 4, ST 44 are used for toothache. The LI channel enters the lower gums and can stop toothaches on the lower jaw. The stomach channel enters the upper gums, St 44 can stop toothaches on the upper jaw.

SI 3 for stiff neck. Because SI 3 is one of the Eight Confluent Points, intersecting with the Du channel. Du channel runs through the neck.

UB 54 for lower back pain, because the UB channel runs through the lower back.

In addition to selecting distal points according to traditional theory, they may also be selected on the basis of nerve distribution. Generally, this is most useful for treatment of disorders of the limb, whereby a point located on a nerve trunk or root above the diseases is selected for needling.

Diseases of the fingers may be treated via points on related nerves. PC 6 on the median nerve near the wrist and LI 11 on the radial nerve near the elbow as well as points on the more distant brachial plexus.

Diseases of the lower limb may be treated at GB 34 on the peroneal nerve and more distally at points along the sciatic nerve or sacral plexus.

Symptomatic point selection

Local and distal points selections are based upon the distance of the points from the site of the diseases. However, some diseases are not local but systemic in nature, and can be treated at points long associated with relieving particular diseases. Prominent among such points are: UB 17 for diseases affecting the blood (the influential point of blood); Ren 17 for diseases of the ch'i (influential point of ch'i); Lu 9 for diseases of the vessels (influential point of vessels); GB 34 for diseases of the tendons (influential point of tendons); GB 39 for diseases of the marrow (influential point of marrow); UB 11 for diseases of the bones (influential point of bones); Liver 13 for diseases of the yin organs, lung, spleen, heart, kidney and liver; Ren 12 for diseases of the yang organs, stomach, large and small intestine, urinary bladder, San Jiao and GB.

Stimulation of these points has proven effective in relieving the disorders with which each is associated. The same is true of the other special point groups. Certain individual points have also traditionally been useful in treating specific symptoms: Du 14 for reducing fever (because Du 14 is the crossing point of the six yang channels and Du Mai); Du 26, for reviving patients from unconsciousness (Du channel enters the brain); pricking and bleeding Lu 11 and SI 1 for sore throat; LI 11, Sp 10, Sp 6 for pruritus (itching); LI 11 cleans wind and heat; Sp 10 and Sp 6 to nourish blood and expel wind evil; Ren 4, St 36, for general weakness. Ren 4 tonifies Yuan source ch'i, and Stomach 36 Tonifies digestive function hence increasing Gu Ch'i.

The efficacy of needling local points to treat disease can be explained not only on the basis of traditional channel theory, but more recently by neural segment theory as well. For example in acupuncture anaesthesia, the point SI 18 is used for surgery on the cranium, and the point LI 18 for operations on the thyroid. Similarly in the clinical treatment of diseases of the viscera, it is common to select a vertebral point on the same horizontal plane as the affected organ. Choosing a point in the same or neighbouring neural segment as that of the pain or disease is also compatible with the rules of traditional local point selection.

In addition to selecting distal points according to traditional theory, they may also be selected on the basis of nerve distribution. Generally, this is most useful for treatment of disorders of the limb, whereby a point located on a nerve trunk or root above the diseases is selected for needling. Diseases of the fingers may be treated via points on related nerves. PC 6 on the median nerve near the wrist and LI 11 on the radial nerve near the elbow as well as points on the more distant brachial plexus. Diseases of the lower limb may be treated at GB 34 on the peroneal nerve and more distally at points along the sciatic nerve or sacral plexus.

Combining points

In addition to the methods of individual point selection outlined above, there are several traditional methods of combining one point with others in an acupuncture prescription. These techniques are flexible, permitting many variations according to the particular needs of the case. The method of combining points on the front (yin aspect of torso) with points on the back (yang aspect of torso) is also known as the combination of abdomen-yin points and the back-yang points. Points on the front and back appropriate to a particular disease can be used in combination. For stomach disease, St 21 on the abdomen and UB 50 on the back could be needled in tandem.

Among the most commonly used front-back combinations are two special point groups, the back-Shu points and the front-Mu points, because these points are closely related to diseases of the Zang Fu organs. For example, one might use Ren 12 (St Front Mu) and UB 21 (Stomach Back Shu) for stomach diseases.

Combining yang and yin channel points

The primary yang channels are connected with the primary yin channels in a yin/yang relationship. By combining a point on a yang channel with another on its paired yin channel, one obtains a greater cumulative effect than by needling either point separately.

Stomach 36 on the yang channel with Sp 4 on the yin channel for stomach diseases. Lung 9 with LI 11, on the paired yang channel, for coughing.

The most well-known combinations of this kind are between the Yuan-source points on the first channel, primarily affected by a disease, and the Luo-connecting point on the paired channel. In this combination the source point is called the 'host', and the connecting point is called the 'guest'.

Diseases affecting the lung channel may be treated through that channel's source point (Lu 9) in combination with the Luo-connecting point (LI 6) of its paired yang partner, the large intestine channel. Conversely, a disease affecting the large intestine channel could be treated by that channel's source point (LI 4), together with the connecting point (Lu 7), of its Yin partner, the lung channel. The method would also encompass the use of a single point, the Luo connecting point of the paired channel.

For a disease associated with the kidney channel, UB 60, the Luo-connecting point of the kidney's paired meridian would be chosen. Conversely, diseases of the UB can be treated by Kidney 4, the Kidney's Luo-connecting point.

Combining points on the left with points on the right

Because channel points are bilateral, it is common to treat diseases of the internal organs by manipulating the same point on both sides in order to strengthen the effect.

UB 21 on both left and right sides of the spine, or St 36 on both legs can be needled to treat diseases of the stomach. Also, because of the intersection of the channels on the right side with those on the left, a point on the right may be chosen to treat a disease of pain on the left side of the body, and vice versa.

In the case of 'stroke,' not only may a point on the side affected by the paralysis be selected, but the same point on the healthy side may be used as well.

Combining points above with points below

Above refers to points on the arms and above the waist (Ren 8). Below refers to points on the legs or below the waist (Ren 8). This method of point combination is most commonly practised on the limbs. In the case of stomach diseases, PC 6 on the arm may be combined with St 36 on the leg. For toothache, LI 4 of the hand can be combined with St 44 on the foot.

Traditionally, a distinctive use of the above–below combination was made with respect to the confluent points of the eight extraordinary channels. A confluent point on an extraordinary channel affected by a disease above would be combined in an acupuncture prescription with a meeting point on an extraordinary channel below.

For diseases of the heart, chest, abdomen, PC 6 on the arm may be combined with Sp 4 on the foot. For ear ringing, SJ 5 on the arm can be combined with GB 41 on the foot.

Combining local with distal points

When there are stomach problems, the local points Ren 12 and UB 21 or the distal points St 36, PC 6 and Sp 4, could be used separately. The combination method, however, uses both the local and distal points together.

Specific points

Specific points are those on the 14 meridians with specific therapeutic significance. Since specific points have different distributions and effects, they have different names. The following represents a brief description of their applications.

The five transporting points (Five Shu)

These are five points on the 12 regular channels, namely the Jing-well, Ying-spring, Shu-stream, Jing-river, and He-sea. The five transporting points may be selected according to their therapeutic properties.

Jing-well points are selected for fullness in the epigastrium (liver/wood element disharmony). Ying-spring points are for febrile diseases (heart/fire element difficulties). Shu-stream points are for a heavy sensation of the body and/or painful joints (spleen/earth element problems). Jing-river points are for cough and asthma due to pathogenic cold or heat (lung/metal element ailments).

He-sea points are for diarrhoea due to rebellious ch'i or Zang organ disharmony (kidney/water element afflictions). This is because the Jing-well points on the yin channels belong to the wood element. Jing-well points on the yang channels belong to the metal element. Because metal controls wood, tonifying the Jing-well points on the yang channels will result in the sedation of liver energy, which is often the needed treatment. Also the Jing-well points on the yin channels can be sedated for a similar effect. Another way to use the Jing-well points that treat more than just the wood element can be found in using PC 9 with K 1. This technique makes use of the above/below combination which, in this case, has the effect of balancing fire (pericardium) and water (kidney), which balances above and below as well as fire and water. Connecting the ch'i of these two opposing elemental forces calms the Shen.

Ying-spring

Ying-spring points are for febrile diseases and heart disharmony. Heart belongs to fire. Febrile diseases are 'fiery'. Signs and symptoms include: irritability and sleeplessness, sores on the tongue and lips, flushed face, thirst, painful and dark coloured urine, dry stool, hematemesis (vomiting blood), nosebleeds, delirium or mania in severe cases, red tongue with yellow coat, rapid pulse.

Again, tonifying the grandmother of fire (water), which is found at the Ying-spring points of the yang channels will sedate the fire element's fire. Sedating the yin channel's Ying-spring (fire) points will help to turn down the fire in the heart or elsewhere.

Shu-stream

Shu-stream points are for spleen diseases, heavy sensations in the body and painful joints due to spleen ch'i deficiency. This Ch'i Xu will also diminish the efficiency of the spleen's function of transportation and transformation. With this hypofunction, dampness will be stored up within the body, or lead to a spleen disorder due to cold-damp retention within the spleen proper. Signs and symptoms include: sensation of fullness in the abdomen, anorexia, nausea and vomiting, weakened limbs, loose stool, pale tongue with white greasy coat, and slow, soft pulse.

Sedating the grandmother of earth (wood) which is found at the Shu-stream points of the yang channels will serve to tonify earth. Tonifying the Shu-stream points on the yin channels will help to build up the strength of the earth element and end the spleen disharmony.

Jing-river

Jing-river points are for lung diseases, cough and asthma due to pathogenic cold or heat. Lungs belong to metal, when lungs are attacked by pathogenic wind-cold or wind-heat, obstruction of the lung ch'i results. Signs and symptoms include: cough, asthma, dry throat, sore throat, hoarseness, and nasal obstruction.

Sedating the grandmother of metal (fire) which is found at the Jing-river points of the yang channels will serve to tonify metal. Tonifying the Jing-river points on the yin channels will help to build up the strength of the metal element and end the metal disharmonies.

He-sea

He-sea points are for kidney diseases and/or diarrhoea due to rebellious ch'i. When the kidney ch'i is deficient, it is unable to grasp the Da ch'i of the lungs. Signs and symptoms include: shortness of breath, dyspnoea, and difficult inhalation (normal exhalation).

Another area affected by kidney ch'i deficiency is that of its reinforcement and astringent functions. Signs and symptoms include: enuresis (withholding of urine), spermatorrhea, diarrhoea, pale tongue with white fur, and a deep and weak pulse. Sedating the grandmother of water (earth) which is found at the He-sea points of the yang channels will serve to tonify water. Tonifying the He-sea points on the yin channels will help to build up the strength of the water element and end the water disharmonies.

Channel	Jing-Well	Ying-Spring	Shu-Stream	Jing-River	He-Sea
Lung	Lu 11	Lu 10	Lu 9	Lu 8	Lu 5
Pericardium	PC 9	PC 8	PC 7	PC 5	PC 3
Heart	H 9	H 8	H 7	H 4	H 3
Spleen (pancreas)	Sp 1	Sp 2	Sp 3	Sp 5	Sp 9
Liver	Lv 1	Lv 2	Lv 3	Lv 4	Lv 8
Kidney	K 1	K 2	K 3	K 7	K 10
Large intestine	LI 1	LI 2	LI 3	LI 5	LI 11
San Jiao	SJ 1	SJ 2	SJ 3	SJ 6	SJ 10
Small intestine	SI 1	SI 2	SI 3	SI 5	SI 8
Stomach	St 45	St 44	St 43	St 41	St 36
Gall bladder	GB 44	GB 43	GB 41	GB 38	GB 34
Urinary bladder	UB 67	UB 66	UB 65	UB 60	UB 40

The five transporting points on the 12 regular channels

How to use transportation points in a mother/son combination for tonifying and sedating

As mentioned earlier, the Jing-well, Ying-spring, Shu-stream, Jing-river and He-sea points of the channels are attributed to the five elements. On the yin channels, the order, from the Jing-well point upward from distal to proximal, is wood, fire, earth, metal, and water. On the yang channels, the order, from the Jing-well point upwards from distal to proximal, is metal, water, wood, fire, earth.

One way in which these points can be used therapeutically is by selecting them according to their relationships in the five element model: inter-promoting (mother to son), interacting (grandmother to grandson), overacting (too much grandmother to grandson), and counteracting (grandson pushing back to grandmother).

Beginning with the relationship of the five elements, each channel has a 'mother' point and a 'son' point. The 'mother point' of a channel has a reinforcing effect on that channel, while the 'son point' has a reducing effect. In the case of an excess condition, one can reinforce the mother and reduce the son on the affected channel. In clinical practice, the two-needle method described above can be used on the mother and son points of the affected channel, or on the points along the mother and son channels.

Mother–son treatment with both points on the affected channel

The liver channel pertains to wood. An excess syndrome of the liver channel can be treated by sedating Liver 2, the fire point on the liver channel. Fire is the son of wood and Liver 2 is the fire point on the liver channel, hence sedating the son will give the mother a chance to settle down from her excess state.

The deficiency state of the liver channel can be treated by tonifying liver 8, because this is the water point on the liver channel, and water is the mother of wood. Liver 8 is the mother point of the Liver channel. This is using the principle of 'tonifying the mother for deficiency syndrome'. Then there is the technique of using the same principle, but on the mother and son channels, rather than the mother and son points on the same channel.

Mother–son treatment with points on the mother or son channel

For an excess syndrome of the liver channel, one would treat the Ying-spring point on the Heart channel (Heart 8), because the heart is the fire channel. That makes it liver's son. Ht 8 is the horary (fire) point on Liver's son channel, hence you are 'sedating the son for excess syndromes'.

Deficiency syndromes of the Liver channel can be treated by tonifying the horary point on the mother channel, which is the kidney. Kidney 10 is the horary point (water point on the water channel). This technique is based on the principle of 'tonifying the mother for deficiency syndromes'.

Mother–son treatments with points based on the interior/ exterior relationship

For a deficiency syndrome of the Liver channel, reinforcing GB 43, the mother point of the GB channel, will tonify wood because GB 43 is the mother point on the yang wood channel.

Excess syndromes of the Liver channel can be treated by reducing GB 38, the son point of the GB channel because GB 38 is the fire point and hence the son point on the yang wood channel.

Back Shu and Front Mu

The Back Shu and Front Mu points are closely related to diseases of the Zang Fu organs. When there is the pathogenic change in the Zang Fu organ, a palpitated reaction to this change, in the form of tenderness or sensitivity, can be detected in the corresponding Back Shu or Front Mu point. Thus, whenever an internal organ is affected, the Back Shu point and the Front Mu points pertaining to that organ may be prescribed either independently or in combination with other specific points, as will be described later on.

Yin diseases of the Zang Fu organs can be treated with Back Shu points. Yin diseases (this includes Zang organ syndromes, deficiency syndromes and cold syndromes) can all be treated with the Back Shu points. Yin diseases reach yang. The evil ch'i of the yin diseases may reach the back Shu points. This is called 'Treating yang for yin diseases'. Another point is 'Lead yin evil out through yang points.' So, needling the Back Shu points to treat yin diseases leads the evil ch'i out through the Back Shu points.

UB 13 on the back is needled to treat productive cough, fullness in the chest, etc., due to yin-type diseases of the lung, in this case, wind cold.

Yang diseases can be treated with the front Mu points. Yang diseases may include Fu organ syndromes, excess syndromes, or heat syndromes. The ch'i of yang diseases may reach the Front Mu points. The treatment principle is then called 'Treating yin for yang diseases'. Leading yang evil out through the yin points we can use the same techniques and needle the Front Mu points.

Ren 3 (the front Mu of the UB) is needled to treat copious, frequent urination, burning pain in the urethra, dark yellow urine, etc., due to damp heat in the UB.

The Back Shu points above (and including) UB 17 can, in addition to the yin diseases described above, treat yang diseases such as exterior cold or heat, chest or back pain (due to lung heat, or wind heat or cold). UB 13 can treat common cold expelling wind heat or wind cold evil. This explains why the Lung Shu point is so versatile for lung or exterior disharmonies. The Front Mu under the level of Ren 8 can treat yin diseases as well as yang in the same way as the Back Shu points above UB 17 can treat yang. For example, Ren 4 can treat leanness due to consumption; ch'i, yang, yin, or Jing collapse; or stroke associated with extreme ch'i, yin, yang, or Jing Xu. The reason

Back Shu points above UB 17 are good for yang diseases as well as yin, is because they are situated on the yang (top half) of the yang aspect of the torso (the back). The are like 'yang within yang' and since 'Ultimate yang becomes yin', they begin to take on the yin functions of treating yang diseases.

The same thing applies to the Front Mu points below the level of Ren 8. They are found on the yin aspect of the body, and the lower, or yin half of the abdomen, and hence they represent 'ultimate yin' which can begin to take on yang attributes and thus treat yin syndromes.

Combining points on the Back Shu with points on the Front Mu

Certain disease syndromes are not simple; they can exhibit signs of both excess and deficiency. In these cases, it is appropriate to use both the Front Mu and Back Shu points.

UB 13 + Lu 1 for lung diseases.
UB 18 + Lv 14 for liver diseases.
UB 19 + GB 24 for gall bladder diseases.
UB 21 + Ren 12 for stomach diseases.
UB 25 + St 25 for large intestine diseases.
UB 28 + Ren 3 for urinary bladder diseases.

Combining Front Mu points with lower He-sea points on the yang channels treats yang diseases (Fu organ syndromes, excess syndromes, heat syndromes). Note: Lower He-sea implies the three extra He-sea points from the hand yang channels as well as the three He-sea points on the foot yang channels as was discussed earlier. For example: St 25 (LI Front Mu) + St 37 (LI Lower He-sea) = treatment of Damp Heat in the large intestine. According to the *Nei Jing*, 'Lower He-sea points treat Fu organ diseases.'

Combining Back Shu points with Yuan-source points treats yin diseases (Zang organ syndromes, deficiency syndromes, cold syndromes). For example: UB 13 (Lung Back Shu) + Lu 9 (Lung Yuan-source point) = treatment of asthma due to lung ch'i deficiency.

UB 23 (Kidney back-Shu) + Kid 3 (Kidney Yuan-source point) = treatment of spermatorrhea due to kidney ch'i deficiency.

Back-Shu points and Yuan-source points can both treat deficiency diseases.

Yuan-source points

The Yuan-source points are located on the six yang channels, and arranged behind the shu-stream points of the five transporting points. On the six yin channels, you'll find the yuan-source points conveniently located directly on the Shu-stream points.

The Yuan-source points are closely related to San Jiao. Acupuncture on the Yuan-source points can dredge the source ch'i in the San Jiao and regulate the functions of the internal organs. Hence Yuan-source points can treat diseases of both the Zang and Fu organs.

Combining Yuan-source points of Zang organs with Yuan-source points of Fu organs

This refers to Yuan-source points of Yang channels on the hand combined with the Yuan-source points of the Yin channels on the foot, or the Yuan-source points of Yin channels on the hand combined with Yuan-source points of Yang channels on the foot.

This technique is beneficial when treating diseases that affect the entire body. Using the hand and foot Yuan-source points together circulates the chi's therapeutic action throughout the entire body. For example: Liver 3 (Yuan-source point of the liver meridian of foot Jue Yin) combines with LI 4, (Yuan-source point of LI meridian of hand Yang Ming) for dizziness, tinnitus, numb limbs and tight tendons due to liver yin deficiency.

Yuan-source points combining with the Luo-connecting points

The Luo-connecting points connect internally, externally related channels. Most beneficial when internally/externally related pairs of channels have a disease together.

Yuan-source points combined with Back Shu points

Back Shu points and Yuan-source points can both treat deficiency diseases. Together, their effects are enhanced.

Yuan-source points combined with He-sea points or lower He-sea points

Interior/Exterior channel relationships. Yuan-source points of yin channels combined with He-sea or lower He-sea points of yang channels. For example: Sp 3 (Yuan-source point of Spleen channel) combined with St 36 (He-sea point of Stomach channel) for abdominal pain, diarrhoea, nausea, and vomiting.

Lv 3 (Yuan-source point of liver channel) combined with GB 34 (He-sea point of GB channel) for dizziness, bitter taste or dryness in the mouth, burning pain in the chest and hypochondrium due to liver or GB fire.

This combination of points (Yuan + He-sea) is used when the cause of the disease is a disharmony between the internally/externally related organs.

Same channel. Yuan-source point combined with He-sea point on the same channel. LI 4 (Yuan-source point of LI channel) combined with LI 11 (He-sea point of LI channel) for headache, toothache, sore throat, dry mouth all due to wind heat evil.

Liver 3 (Yuan-source) combined with Liver 8 (He-sea) for distension. Cramping and cold pain in the perineum and lower abdomen, or pain from contraction of the scrotum due to accumulation of cold in the Liver channel. Different channels, not internally/externally related. LI 4 combined with St 36 regulates stomach and LI for treatment of dry stool.

LI 4 to tonify Jin (as in Jin/Ye) and St 36 tonifies the stomach to push the faecal matter out of the intestines.

Liver 3 combined with St 36. Disperses stagnated liver ch'i, regulates stomach ch'i, for treatment of stomach ache due to liver ch'i stagnation. Regulates liver ch'i and tonifies earth that has been attacked by wood.

Luo-connecting points

The Luo-connecting points are closely related to collaterals. A Luo-connecting point connects with its partner in the interior/exterior relationship. That's why the Luo-connecting points are indicated in the syndromes of their partners in the interior/exterior relationship. For instance Spleen 4, the Luo-connecting point of the Spleen channel of Foot Tai Yin, can treat not only the diseases of the spleen channel, but also those of the stomach channel. Lu7, the Luo-connecting point of the lung channel of Hand Tai Yin can treat not only the diseases of the lung channel (cough, asthma), but also those of the LI channel (toothache, head and neck diseases).

As for Du 1, Ren 15, and Sp 21 (the Luo-connecting point of the so-called 'Greater Collateral of the Spleen, rules collaterals and blood vessels), they are mainly selected to treat their respective diseased parts and disorders of the internal organs.

The Eight Confluent points of the extra meridians

The *Yi Xue Ru Men* (Introduction to Medicine) says that 'among the 360 points on the whole body, 66 points located at the four extremities are important, and among these 66 points, the Eight Confluent points are considered the most important.'

The Eight Confluent points are the points where the extra meridians connect to the 12 primary meridians. There are four Luo-connecting points among the eight confluent points. They are PC 6, Sp 4, SJ 5, Lu 7, and two Shu-stream points which are SI 3 and GB 41. (UB 62, K 6 have no function other than their connections to the Eight Extras – Yin Qiao Mai and Yang Qiao Mai.) In practice, the eight confluent points of extra meridians may be used independently:

Sp 4 for diseases of the spleen, stomach and Chong Mai.
PC 6 for diseases of the pericardium, heart, San Jiao and Yin Wei Mai.
Lu 7 for diseases of the lung, large intestine and Ren Mai.
K 6 for diseases of the kidney and Yin Qiao Mai.
SJ 5 for diseases of the San Jiao, pericardium and Yang Wei Mai.
GB 41 for diseases of the gall bladder and Dai Mai.
SI 3 for diseases of the small intestine and Du Mai.
UB 62 for diseases of the urinary bladder and Yang Qiao Mai.

The confluent points on the upper limb can be combined with the confluent points on the lower limb:

Sp 4 is combined with PC 6 for specific treatment of heart, chest, and stomach disease.
Lu 7 is combined with K 6 for specific treatment of lung, chest, throat and diaphragm disease.
SJ 5 is combined with GB 41 for specific treatment of outer canthus, ear, shoulder, neck or cheek disease.
SI 3 is combined with UB 62 for specific treatment of inner canthus, nape and shoulder disease.

Xi-cleft points

Each of the 12 regular channels has one Xi-cleft point. In addition one Xi-cleft point can be found on each of Yin Wei, Yang Wei, Yin Qiao, Yang Qiao channels. There are 16 Xi-cleft points in all. They are used primarily in treatment of the acute pain and diseases appearing in their corresponding channels and organs. Xi-cleft on the yin channels can stop bleeding. For example: Lu 6 for hemoptysis; Sp 8 for menorrhagia. Xi-cleft on the yang channels can stop pain. For example: LI 7 for toothache, sore throat, headache. St. 34 is used for stomach ache.

Lower He-sea points

The disorders of the Six Fu organs can be treated by the He-sea points. According to this theory, the lower He-sea points are selected to treat diseases of their respective Fu organs. For instance: dysentery and appendicitis are treated by St 37, because St 37 is the lower He-sea point of the LI channel. UB 39 is used for retention of urine due to dysfunction of San Jiao.

Crossing points

These are points located at the intersection of two or more channels. The channels that cross can be primary, extraordinary, or both. They can be used to treat disorders of each of their pertaining channels. They are often used to treat the diseases simultaneously in meridians intersecting each other.

Sp 6, a crossing point for the three foot yin channels, is used for diseases of the liver, spleen and kidney channels.

Finding a practitioner

Currently in the United States there are some 8,000 licensed acupuncturists, about 6,000 of whom prescribe Chinese herbs. In addition there are about 4,000 medical doctors who practise acupuncture; most of these do not prescribe Chinese herbs. There are also over a thousand other health professionals, mainly naturopathic physicians, nutritionists, massage therapists, and chiropractors who prescribe Chinese herbs but do not perform acupuncture.

Over a third of these practitioners completed their training during the last five years. The others received their training between 1975 and 1990. The majority of practitioners of Chinese medicine live in just nine states: California, Washington, Oregon, New Mexico, Colorado, Texas, New York, Massachusetts and Florida. Most of them live in and around major cities.

To find a practitioner of Chinese medicine may not always be easy. If you don't know anyone who can give you a personal recommendation try looking in the yellow pages of your phone directory (or that of the nearest major city) for acupuncturists, for Chinese herbalists, or similar headings for the other types of practitioners.

You will need to call and find out what sort of treatment they practise as well as what sort of training they have had. Your herbalist (who may also be your acupuncturist) should have either a certificate of training or a long-standing reputation and years of experience. Many schools train people in herbal medicine, but there is no independent licensing for Chinese herbalists in the UK or USA. California is the only state that requires practitioners to take an exam in both acupuncture and herbal therapy to be licensed to practise acupuncture. The NCCA does offer a herbal certification, but it doesn't lead to licensing.

If you are looking for a primary care physician, find someone who is knowledgeable about all aspects of Chinese medicine and Western medical procedures; someone who will know when to refer you for Western evaluations and testing, and who is willing to work with a Western doctor if doing so provides you with the best therapy.

To sum up what to look for in a primary care Chinese medicine practitioner:

- Someone who does not make promises to cure incurable diseases (applies to all practitioners, no matter what you use them for);
- Someone who understands that there may be many different modalities that work for an individual and does not insist that their way is the only right or good way to go;
- Someone whose bedside manner pleases you. (Some people don't care about personality; for others, a more personal relationship is important.)
- Someone who is able to explain procedures from both a Chinese and a Western viewpoint, or is at least willing to find out about the alternative perspective when necessary;

- Someone who is not unconditionally opposed to any drug therapy in conjunction with acupuncture or herbal treatment, and who understands the interactions of drugs and herbs;
- Someone who will work with Western medical doctors and other practitioners;
- In cases of serious illnesses, someone who understands Western medical terminology and concepts of the immune system, viruses and cancer, as well as Chinese concepts.

Receiving treatment

When you select a practitioner and go for treatment, you don't surrender control of your health. Chinese medicine recognises that we each possess the means we need to preserve or reclaim good health. The experienced practitioner simply acts as the catalyst, helping to coax the body's own defences to prevent or repair ill health.

There are four basic healing techniques that the practitioner may suggest as treatments: acupuncture and moxibustion, herbal therapy, dietary therapy, and Ch'i Kung exercise/meditation. Only a brief description is given below, as each therapy is discussed in detail elsewhere in this book.

Dietary therapy

Chinese dietary therapy uses foods to strengthen digestion, increase energy and balance the body's energy. Dietary therapy is often used prior to or in conjunction with other therapies to increase the effectiveness of these treatments.

Acupuncture and moxibustion

Classic acupuncture is the art of inserting fine, sterile, metal needles into certain points along the channels and collaterals (tributaries of the channels) in order to control the flow of ch'i. These days, practitioners also use electro-stimulation of the needles, lasers and even ultrasound to stimulate the points.

Acupuncture is well known for its effectiveness as a painkiller. Even more powerful is its ability to alter the flow of the ch'i so that the body can heal itself when attacked by pathogens that trigger disharmony. Acupressure and massage are closely related to acupuncture.

Moxibustion, the burning of the herb *Artemisia vulgaris* (Chinese or common mugwort) over channel points and certain areas of the body, is used to warm, tonify and stimulate. It also induces the smooth flow of the Essential Substances, prevents diseases and preserves health. Doing moxibustion regularly on specific acupuncture points is said to promote strength and longevity.

Chinese herbal medicine

Although the overwhelming majority of medicinal substances come from plants, some are derived from minerals and animals. Whatever their origin, they are used to balance the overall body as well as to reverse disease processes. Most Chinese herbs should only be taken under the supervision of a trained herbalist.

Ch'i Kung

Ch'i Kung, the Chinese art of exercise, uses dynamic movements and still postures in combination with mental and spiritual concentration to influence the flow of ch'i. It is a powerful preventative therapy and can help remedy disharmony in the organ systems and the channels.

6

ACUPRESSURE

*Heaven is long-enduring and earth continues long. The reason
why heaven and earth are able to endure and continue thus long is
because they do not live of, or for, themselves. This is how they are
able to continue and endure.*

Tao Ti Ching

How acupressure works

The science of acupressure and acupuncture is based on a theory that is
totally different from allopathic (i.e. Western) medicine. The theory
states that the human body has various meridians that carry energy
throughout the body. These meridians start at the fingertips, connect to
the brain, and then connect to the organ associated with the specific
meridian. The names of these meridians specify the organ associated
with them. For example, the lung meridian is connected to the lungs
via the nervous system. Theoretically, a lung problem arises if there is
an obstruction in the lung meridian that slows down the flow of energy.
If somehow the obstruction is removed or dissolved, the energy flow
becomes regular and the lungs start functioning well. In acupressure
the meridian is stimulated by pressure rather than by needles.

One interesting theory states that it is not necessarily the organ that
relates to the system that causes the problem. It is the 'root cause' that
is the main cause of the disease/malfunction and if the root problem is
cured, the external problem is cured as well. This can be explained in
an easier way by using an example. Suppose a person is suffering from
asthma. An allopathic doctor would prescribe a medicine such as a

steroid, that would give rest to the lungs and relieve the symptoms because an allopathic doctor thinks that the cause for asthma problems is in the lungs. An acupressurist, on the other hand, will try to find the root cause – the reason why the lungs are malfunctioning. An acupressurist reads the whole body by reading energy pulses located on the arms to diagnose the root cause, and then attempts to cure that specific problem, rather than the asthma. A root cause could be anything like poor digestion, excessive heat, bad circulation, depression, or bad hormones. It could even be the organ itself. So it could be that the asthmatic's lungs are the root cause of the problem.

─────── Using acupressure ───────

Acupressure points on the back of the hand and examples of their function

1 Loin and leg. Sciatica and low back pain especially in acute stage.
2 Ankle. Sprained ankle, rheumatic pain.
3 Chest. Intercostal neuritis, vomiting, epilepsy.
4 Eye. Acute conjunctivitis.
5 Shoulder. Frozen shoulder.
6 Forehead. Frontal headaches, abdominal pain, gastro-enteritis.
7 Vertex. Headache.
8 Unilateral half of head. Right- or left-sided headache, chest pain, biliary colic.
9 Perineum. Pain in perianal region.
10 Occiput. Posterior headache, acute tonsillitis, arm pain, hiccough.
11 Vertebral column. Low back pain, tinnitus, rhinitis.
12 Sciatic nerve. Sciatica, hip pain.
13 Throat. Tonsillitis, pharyngitis, toothache, trigeminal neuralgia.
14 Neck and nape. Cervical syndrome.
15 Nasal bleeding. Epistaxis.
16 Head. Headache.
17 Nasal pain. Sinusitis.
18 Wrist pain. Sprained wrist.

Acupressure points on the palm of the hand and examples of their function

19 GI tract. Abdominal pain, gasto-enteritis.

20 Heel. Sprained ankle.
21 Common cold. Influenza, rhinitis.
22 Hysteria. Emotional disturbance.
23 Cough, sore throat, chronic bronchitis.
24 Oral ulcer, mouth pain.
25 Palpitations, dizziness, chest discomfort.
26 Nocturia. Kidney diseases.
27 Nocturia. Bed-wetting.
28 Polyhidrosis. Excessive sweating.
29 Lung. Chronic cough, chest discomfort.
30 Large intestine. Vomiting, abdominal pain.
31 Small intestine. Diarrhoea.
32 Heart palpitation.
33 San-chiao. Lymphatic disorders.
34 Spleen. Blood diseases.
35 Liver. Jaundice, indigestion.
36 Toothache.

The above only covers a selection of acupressure points. Any appropriate acupressure point on the body can be used, which is especially useful in an emergency if no other means of treatment is available. Acupressure can also be used to complement any conventional treatment to speed up healing.

Acupressure can be used to relieve the symptoms of many illnesses and disorders. If you want to study it further, please see the Further Reading list at the end of the book. In the meantime here a few ways in which acupressure can be used.

Acupressure pain control

If you ever suffer from pain – for example in the neck or back – there's a self-help remedy you'll want to learn: it works almost instantly and requires only a few minutes of training to master the basics. This ancient Chinese technique uses no drugs or medications, only your fingertip. This safe and effective method can be used by nearly anyone to replace aspirin or other common remedies as well as to complement standard Western first-aid methods and procedures.

Acupressure is used symptomatically – that is, as soon as the pain is noticed. It is applied in the same way for both acute problems (e.g. an occasional 'pinched nerve' or 'crick' in the neck) and chronic (more long-standing) disorders, or under emergency conditions – for example, following a road accident. However, there may be a difference in the number of times the technique is applied. For acute problems, if you need to use acupressure more than four or five times during a day, or for more than several days in a row for an apparently minor problem, you're probably using the wrong technique or the wrong pressure point (there are at least a dozen of these tiny pressure points for relief of distress in the neck).

In chronic or emergency use, you may need to apply acupressure a greater number of times in the beginning of self-treatment (maybe several dozen times or more in the first day or two). But in every case, use common sense. If the symptom persists, it may be more serious than you suspect and professional help is advised.

This remarkably effective technique – a mainstay of Chinese families for thousands of years – is a simple, three-step process. Step one is to find the acupressure point that 'controls' the neck area. This is done by probing deeply – as deeply as you can (up to 20 lb of fingertip pressure) – in the general area where the point is located.

Use the tip of the thumb (if you have long nails, the bent knuckle of the index finger or the eraser end of a pencil will work equally well), and probe until you contact a tender 'ouch point'. It should feel like a toothache or pinched nerve when you find it. But since the points are tiny (only about the size of a pinhead), you must use specific pressure. If you miss the spot by even a quarter of an inch, this technique won't be effective. And the sensitivity you'll feel when you contact the spot is the primary way you'll know you've found it.

Step two is to trigger the spot deeply. Do it in a digging, goading kind of fingertip massage. The more sensitive and tender the point, the more likely it is to be a good control point. If it makes you feel warm, break out in a sheen of perspiration or feel a bit light-headed, so much the better. These phenomena are called 'acupressure reactions' and usually occur with the right triggering of a good point. Do this deep stimulation for about 15–30 seconds, then stop.

Step three is to trigger the identical spot on the opposite side of the body (nearly always, these points are duplicated bilaterally – that is, on either side of the body). Then 'test' your symptom. It should be gone, or nearly so. If there's a bit of discomfort remaining, go back and trigger that pair of points again. If the pain is gone, stop.

An acupressure point should be triggered for a maximum of four minutes. If you get no relief by then, it's probably the wrong point (or no point at all), or else you haven't triggered it properly. Reread these instructions and try once more. If acupressure doesn't relieve the discomfort completely, it's usually because you've used the wrong point. Then it's time to try the next point. Simply do the same three-step process – probe, trigger, test – and stop when you obtain relief.

There are some people who should normally avoid the use of acupressure (except for an emergency or limited-time use) before checking with their doctors. These include chronic heart sufferers, especially those wearing pacemakers or other mechanical regulators, and people who take regular, daily medications for serious health problems (cancer, diabetes, etc.).

Pregnant women should also avoid the use of acupressure, especially after the third month of pregnancy. However, there are a couple of very effective acupressure points for use during and following delivery (Points #5, #7 and #13). These pressure points speed the procedure and the subsequent healing process.

As with any self-health technique, follow the same guidelines as you would for non-prescription medicines: if pain or symptoms persist, see your doctor or other health care professional.

Neck tension or injury

Begin with acupressure point #4. Place your right hand so the palm is facing down. Then bend it back slightly so that a crease appears at your wrist. Remember where this crease is, and relax your hand.

Now measure the width of two left thumbs (about two inches) back from that crease towards your elbow, and begin pressing very deeply between the two arm bones (the radius and ulna), in line with the middle finger. You're probing for the small hollow or depression between these two bones.

Once you find the tender spot, follow step two: trigger the point in the manner described above. Finally, duplicate the process on your left forearm.

Then test your symptoms. Your neck should be virtually free of pain or discomfort. If so, but your symptoms later return, simply duplicate the same technique.

If acupressure point #4 fails to work, try point #116. Press about two inches down from your elbow (toward your hand) on the outside (hairy side) of your upper forearm. Probe deeply in the muscle until you feel a very tender spot – that's #116. It will be quite tender with even moderate pressure – in fact it's a judo disabling point. Trigger and test as described above.

Both points #4 and #116 work for a broad range of ailments, particularly those in the hands, elbows, arms and shoulders, so you may notice unexpected benefits there as well, after having triggered the point or points.

Pre-menstrual tension

There are over 20 known pressure points to relieve the various symptoms of PMT, and three of the most basic often 'overlap' in their span of effectiveness. Nearly always one will succeed in bringing prompt relief. If you try one point and don't get results, try another.

Upon finding and triggering a good point properly, several things usually occur. First, you'll often feel a sudden sense of warmth or perspiration. Even a sense of light-headedness or, rarely, a brief touch of nausea. These are perfectly normal acupressure reactions and simply serve to indicate you've triggered one of the better points for your problem. Then, after a few seconds of massage, check your PMT symptoms. They should be nearly or totally gone. If you've applied acupressure properly, you should get near-total relief. Suffering often vanishes completely and immediately, as if it had never existed.

To find acupressure point #7, measure the width of one hand (about three inches) up from the bony bulge of the inner ankle (medial malleolus). The point is found alongside the shinbone (tibia), or in the space between the shinbone and calf muscle.

For acupressure point #9, measure one hand-width below the bottom of the kneecap. Slightly to the outside (lateral side, direction of the little toe) of the ridge of the shinbone, you should discover a long, vertical trough or valley separating the shinbone and the front of the calf muscle. Acupressure point #9 is found in that depression.

Acupressure point #10 is found by measuring two thumbs (roughly two inches) above the most prominent crease of the inner wrist (direction of the elbow), in line with your middle finger. Probe between the tendons in your lower forearm. The point should ache when you contact it – not twinge sharply as some other points (notably #7) might.

Dieting

The Chinese use this acupressure technique when they're dieting. Next time you're hungry, squeeze your earlobes for one minute. At the very least, it will keep your hands busy until the craving passes.

Staying awake

Here's an experiment that proves you can keep your eyes open even under the most exhausting circumstances. This comes in handy whenever keeping your eyes open and yourself alert is necessary to avoid embarrassment or injury.

1 Sit back in your chair with your feet (both of them) squarely on the floor. If you've been clutching a briefcase, clipboard or purse, put it on the table or floor.
2 Put your hands in your lap. With your right thumb, dig deep into the middle of the palm of your left hand. Hold for one minute.
3 Reverse and dig your left thumb into your right palm.
4 Now pinch the base of each finger tightly. Hold each for about 30 seconds.
5 Repeat with the other hand.
6 Now press with your thumb on the outer edge of your forearm at about two-inch intervals all the way up to the elbow on one side.
7 Now continue on the other side back down to the wrist.
8 Do the same with the other arm.

These are only a few simple tips. If you want to learn more, see the Further Reading list at the end of the book.

7

CONDITIONS TREATED

(The Tao) produces (all things) and nourishes them; it produces them and does not claim them as its own; it does all, and yet does not boast of it; it presides over all, and yet does not control them. This is what is called 'The mysterious Quality' (of the Tao).

Tao Ti Ching

Chinese medical diagnosis is very different from the Western variety, as is the Chinese classification of disorders and diseases. For instance you wouldn't expect a Chinese practitioner to diagnose cancer, but rather blood Xu (blood stagnation). This chapter covers some of the most common types of diagnosis and treatment.

Aversion to wind and cold along with chills

The difference between chills and aversion to cold is that chills are not eased or relieved by warm clothing whereas aversion to cold is. In 99 per cent of cases this is an exterior syndrome. The three exterior forms are dealt with first.

Fever and chills caused by wind, though it can be combined with other factors

Symptoms: Muscle aches, headache. Wind with cold. Chills and aches. *Formula*: Ma Huang Tang (Pungent and warm).

Wind with heat

Symptoms: Fever and sore throat. *Formula*: Yin Ch'iao San (Pungent and cool).

Wind with damp

Symptoms: Stuffiness, aching in joints. *Formula*: Ch'ian Wei Ch'iang Hua.

Internal yin (warm and dry) conditions are dealt with next.

Yang collapse (kidney and heart most affected)

Symptoms: Feeble or faint pulse. Very low energy. Confusion and disorientation. Cold sweat, cold body, cold extremities. Low blood-pressure. Patient prefers foetal position. Diarrhoea with undigested food. Clear, copious urine. *Treatment*: Restore yang from collapse. *Formula*: Shen Fu Tang.

Yang Xu (not as severe as collapse) (heart, spleen, kidney)

Symptoms: Aversion to cold. Fatigue. Ch'i Xu. Sx + Cold Sx. Heart yang Xu. Palpitations, fatigue, cyanosis. *Formula*: Gui Zhi Tang with more Zhi Gan Cao. Spleen yang Xu, add Li Zhong Tang. Kidney yang Xu add Jin Gui Shen Ch'i Tang, also known as Ba Wei Di Huang Wan.

True Heat, Pseudo Cold

(An excess condition due to a variety of causes which pushes the yin from the interior to the superficial)

Symptoms: Cold Sx externally. Aversion to cold. Cold skin (which warms upon prolonged touch). Warm Sx internally. Doesn't desire warm clothes. Bad breath, constipation. *Tongue*: Red with yellow coat. *Pulse*: Forceful and rapid. *Formula*: Bai Hu Tang.

Phlegm accumulation

(Yin evil blocks the flow of yang energy, leading to aversion to cold)

Symptoms: Thirst, with no desire to drink. Aversion to cold. *Tongue*: Thick, greasy white coat. *Pulse*: Slippery. *Formula*: Er Chen Tang.

Alternating fever and chills

Shao yang disease

Symptoms: Bitter taste in mouth. Dry mouth. Chest and hypochondriac discomfort. Irritability. *Tongue*: Red tip with thin yellow coat. *Pulse*:

Wiry. *Treatment*: 'Harmonise interior and exterior', which means disperse exterior and clear interior. *Formula*: Xiao Chai Hu Tang.

Malaria

Symptoms: Very regular cycle between fever and chills. Patient is very weak and needs to sleep after each cycle. *Formula*: Ch'ing Hao and Zhong San herbs.

Aversion to heat without chills

(Interior excess condition affecting the lung and stomach)

Hot phlegm in lung (pneumonia, bronchitis)

Symptoms: Fever. Cough. Chest pain. Sputum is thick and yellow, brown, or green. Thirst. Constipation. One can remove heat from lungs by purging constipation. *Tongue*: Red with thick, greasy yellow coat. *Pulse*: Rapid and slippery. *Formula*: Ma Xing Shi Gan Tang.

Yang Ming Jing (Stomach channel)

(No chills because the pathogen is too far interior)

Symptoms: Thirst, fever, sweating, large pulse. *Formula*: Bai Hu Tang (Bitter and cold).

Yang Ming Fu (Large Intestine organ)

Symptoms: Heat leads to fever. Constipation. Bloating. Palpable hardness in abdomen (dry stool). *Pulse*: Deep, strong, slow (slow due to stagnation). *Formula*: Da Cheng Ch'i Tang.

Ying or Xue level syndromes (pericardium)

Symptoms: High fever (104 degrees F and above). Mental manifestations (confusion, delirium, etc.). *Tongue*: Red with scanty, or no coat (yin deficiency). *Formula*: herbs include Xi Jiao, Ling Yang Jiao and Shui Niu Jiao.

Tidal fever (low-grade fever)

Yin Xu

Symptoms: Low-grade fever in the afternoon or evening. Five centre heat. *Formula*: Liu Wei Di Huang Wan. Ch'i Xu (Spleen/Stomach Ch'i Xu). *Symptoms*: Low-grade fever at no regular time. Fever + Ch'i Xu symptoms. *Formula*: Bu Zhong Yi Ch'i Tang.

Blood stagnation

(Late stage stagnation leads to blood Xu, as in late-stage cancer) *Symptoms*: Low-grade fever in evening. Aches. Dry skin. Dark circles under eyes. Tumour formation. *Tongue*: Purple. *Pulse*: Choppy and thready. *Treatment:* Remove blood stagnation.

Yang Ming Fu syndrome (large intestine)

Symptoms: Low fever possible, due to stagnation. Fever. Constipation. *Formulas*: Da Ching Ch'i Tang, or any of the related 'Ching Ch'i Tang' formulas.

Five centre heat

Yin deficiency with deficiency heat

Symptoms: Five centre heat, which is heat manifesting on the yin surfaces of the body, such as the palms, bottom of the feet, and the chest. Night sweats, hot flushes. *Tongue*: Red, narrow, scanty coat. *Pulse*: Thin and rapid. *Treatment*: Nourish yin, remove heat. *Formula*: Liu Wei Di Huang Wan (tonifies yin). Zhi Bai Di Huang Wan (clears deficiency heat). *Important herbs*: Huang Bai, Zhi Mu. Bitter and cold, they cool both deficiency and excess heat.

Blood deficiency leading to deficiency heat (liver/spleen)

Symptoms: Five centre heat especially in the afternoon and evening. Fatigue, poor appetite, palpitations, dizziness, vertigo, pale complexion. *Tongue*: Pale. *Pulse*: Thready, soft, or choppy. *Treatment*: Nourish blood. *Formula*: Si Wu Tang.

Night sweats (sweat is the fluid of the heart)

Heart blood deficiency

Symptoms: Night sweats. Palpitations, insomnia, pale complexion, fatigue. *Tongue*: Pale. *Pulse*: Weak. *Treatment*: Tonify heart blood, astringent sweat. *Formula*: Si Wu Tang, plus an astringent such as Wu Wei Zi, Long Gu, My Li, Fu Xiao Mai, Gui Pi Tang.

Yin deficiency with deficiency heat

Symptoms: Night sweats. Palpitations, insomnia, pale complexion fatigue. *Tongue*: Pale. *Pulse*: Weak. *Treatment*: Tonify yin. *Formula*: Liu Wei Di Huang Wan + astringent such as Fu Xiao Mai.

Obesity

Accumulation of phlegm and damp (excess condition)

Symptoms: Obesity, excess appetite. Likes sweet and fatty, greasy food. Heavy sensations in body, foggy thinking. Aversion to heat. *Tongue*: Flabby; thick, greasy coat. *Pulse*: Wiry/slippery. Wiry can suggest phlegm, heat, or food stagnation. Left untreated, the phlegm can lead to heat, leading to yin deficiency, leading to wind, leading to stroke. *Treatment*: Remove damp and phlegm. *Formula*: Wen Dan Tang + Ping Wei San. These formulas are combined to lose weight; more gentle and safe than Ma Huang based formulas.

Ch'i deficiency (deficiency condition)

Symptoms: Fatigue, weak voice, shortness of breath. Phlegm damp accumulation. Aversion to cold, oedema, puffy face, poor digestion, sleepy. Not necessarily an overeating problem. *Tongue*: Pale with white coating. *Pulse*: Thready and weak. *Treatment*: Tonify yang, raise metabolism.

Emaciation

Spleen/stomach deficiency (stressed digestive problems)

Symptoms: Anaemia, malnutrition, indigestion, thin constitution with indigestion. Poor appetite, chronic loose stool, fatigue, shortness of breath, weak voice. Sallow or pale complexion. *Tongue*: Pale. *Pulse*: Weak. *Treatment*: Tonify spleen. *Formula*: Si Jun Zi Tang. Ba Zhen Tang. Stress carminative herbs.

Ch'i and blood deficiency (digestive problems less stressed)

Symptoms: Anaemia, malnutrition. Pale face, nails, tongue, lips.

Fatigue, dizziness, vertigo. Yang ch'i and blood unable to rise to nourish head. *Tongue*: Pale. *Pulse*: Thready/weak. *Formula*: Ba Zhen Tang. Stress tonic herbs such as He Shou Wu, E Jiao, Ji Xue Teng.

Lung yin deficiency

(Any yin deficiency leads to a certain amount of emaciation)

Symptoms: Thin, emaciated body. Chronic dry cough, i.e. allergies. Lung TB, AIDS, both lead to this sort of emaciation. Cough with blood-streaked sputum. Hematemesis. Dry mouth, tidal fever, night sweats, five centre heat. *Tongue*: Red with scanty coat. *Pulse*: Thready, rapid. *Treatment*: Tonify yin. *Formula*: Bai He Gu Jin Tang for Lung Yin deficiency. Liu Wei Di Huang Wan for any yin deficiency.

Stomach heat (genetic, or acquired, usually chronic)

Symptoms: Excessive appetite, hypermetabolism, bad breath, thin constitution. Craves cold drinks. Irritability. Scanty urine, tends to be constipated. *Tongue*: Red with dry coat. *Pulse*: Thready, rapid, forceful. *Formula*: Jing Wei Tang for stomach heat; Yu Niu Jiao for stomach yin deficiency due to stomach heat.

Liver fire (excess heat)

Symptoms: Easily angered. Chest and hypochondriac pain or burning. Bitter taste, dry mouth. Insomnia, restlessness. Dark yellow urine, constipation. *Tongue*: Red with yellow coat. *Pulse*: Wiry, rapid, forceful. *Formula*: Long Dong Xie Gan Tang.

Fatigue

Summer heat

(Often associated with damp, because the heat weakens the spleen, leading to production of damp)

Symptoms: Symptoms follow excessive sweating, sunstroke, always involved with climatological exposure to heat. Fatigue and weakness in extremities. Dehydration, shortness of breath. Fever. Weak voice, thirst. Dusky face colour if damp is involved. Possible loose stool. *Tongue*: Possible greasy coat. *Pulse*: Weak and rapid, may be soft. *Formula*: Ch'ing Su Yi Ch'i Tang.

Accumulation of damp

(Could be associated with a spleen deficiency if the symptoms stress it)

Symptoms: Sluggish and heavy sensations. Cloudy, foggy head. Spleen ch'i deficiency. Indigestion, loose stool, bloating, low appetite. *Tongue*: Greasy coat. *Pulse*: Soft and slippery. *Treatment*: Dry damp, stimulate digestion. *Formula*: Ping Wei San. Then later, tonify spleen.

Ch'i and blood deficiency

Symptoms: Fatigue and pale skin, face, lips, nails, etc. Dizziness, palpitations. *Tongue*: Pale. *Pulse*: Deep, thready, weak. *Formula*: Ba Zheng Tang.

Flaccidity of neck and head

(Due to weakened muscles; a serious condition wherein the patient is unable to raise the head)

Zhong Ch'i Xu

(More often affects children with sever malnutrition, Jing deficiency, Down's syndrome)

Symptoms: Severe emaciation. Pale or sallow complexion. Disorientation, confusion, extreme fatigue. Indigestion, loose stool. Middle Jiao deficiency leads to Zhong deficiency.

Bone marrow deficiency (critical condition)

Symptoms: Comes due to old age, sexual hyperactivity, associated with tinnitus, low back pain, difficulty in walking or straightening back. *Tongue*: Pale with scanty coating. *Pulse*: Deep, very weak, or feeble. *Treatment*: Tonify kidney Jing. *Formulas*: Herbs made of animal products to quickly tonify.

Involuntary twitching of head muscles

Liver wind, liver fire (acute excess condition)

Symptoms: Twitching, acute, dizziness, bodily twitches in extremities especially. Red face, eyes, bitter taste in mouth. *Tongue*: Red with yellow coat. *Pulse*: Rapid and wiry. *Formula*: Ling Jiao Gou Teng Tang – removes wind, clears heat.

Liver wind (chronic deficiency condition – Parkinson's disease)

Symptoms: Tidal fever, night sweats, insomnia, fatigue. *Tongue*: Red with scanty coat. *Pulse*: Thready and rapid. *Treatment*: Tonify yin, soothe liver, disperse wind. *Formula*: Da Ding Feng Zhu.

Tinnitus cranii (noise in the head)

Bone marrow deficiency

Symptoms: Tinnitus. Weakness/soreness in the lower back and/or knees. Vertigo/dizziness. Possibly associated with ear tinnitus. *Tongue*: Pale with scanty coat. *Pulse*: Deep, thready, weak. *Causes*: Constitution, age, over-sexed, Jing deficiency fails to produce Jing. *Treatment*: Tonify Jing. *Formula*: Zhou Gui Wan. He Che Da Zao Wan. Animal products are good for Jing Xu.

Damp heat accumulation

Symptoms: Tinnitus. Headache, heavy sensation in head. Nausea/vomiting. Poor appetite. Dizziness. Chuan Yang (carbuncles on head). *Tongue*: Red with greasy yellow coat. *Pulse*: Slippery, rapid. *Causes*: Excess conditions due to diet of sweet, greasy, alcohol, or over-indulgence creates damp heat in channels which obstructs the flow of yang ch'i. Obstruction in upper Jiao affects the head channels. *Treatment*: Clear heat, dry damp. *Formula*: Huang Lian Jie Tu Tang plus blood activators for sharp fixed pain.

Liver ch'i stagnation

Symptoms: Tinnitus triggered by anger or emotion. Distension or pain in the hypochondrium, chest tightness. Bitter taste in mouth. Irritability, restlessness. *Tongue*: Normal. *Pulse*: Wiry and rapid. *Causes*: Anger leads to disturbance in flow of ch'i, leads to stagnation of ch'i in the head. *Treatment*: Soothe liver ch'i. *Formula*: Xiao Yao Wan. Long Dan Xie Gan Tang if Fire is present.

Sore gums

Deficiency of kidney and spleen (teeth and gums)
Symptoms: Sore gums aggravated mostly by cold drinks and weather,

sometimes hot drinks as well. Teeth feel weak while chewing. *Tongue*: Pale. *Pulse*: Deep and weak. *Causes*: Old age, chronic conditions. *Treatment*: Tonify spleen and kidney. *Formula*: Zuo Gui Yin. Ruo Gui Yin. Liu Wei Di Huang Wan. Ba Wei Di Huang Wan. Chew and eat walnuts (Hu Tao Ren).

Wind cold

Symptoms: Sore gums, prefer warm drinks and food to cold. *Tongue*: White, slippery coat (slightly greasy). *Pulse*: Floating and tense. *Formula*: Xi Xin (individual herb) can be chewed raw, or decocted as a tea. Ma Huang Xi Xin Fu Zi Tang.

Bleeding gums (ulcerative gingivitis)

Heat and fire in stomach/large intestine (excess condition, acute)

Symptoms: Swollen, red aching bleeding gums. Fresh, bright red blood. Bad breath, prefers cold drinks, constipation. *Tongue*: Red body, thick yellow coat. *Pulse*: Forceful and rapid. *Formula*: Ch'ing Wei Tang + Yu Niu Jiao + herbs to cool and activate blood.

Stomach yin deficiency (deficiency condition, chronic)

Symptoms: Swollen gums with pale blood, gums not bright red, sometimes painful, sometimes not. *Tongue*: Red with scanty coat. *Pulse*: Slippery, rapid, thready. *Formula*: Yu Niu Jiao + herbs to cool and activate blood.

Kidney yin deficiency with excess heat (chronic condition associated with old age)

Symptoms: Slightly sore gums combined with loose teeth. Dizziness, tinnitus. Sore back and weak knees. *Tongue*: Red body with scanty coat. *Pulse*: Thready and rapid. *Formulas*: (with heat) Zhi Bei Di Huang + Gu Sui Bu and/or Xu Duan; (without heat) Rou Gui Yin or Zuo Gui Yin + Gu Sui Bu and/or Xu Duan.

Spleen ch'i deficiency (spleen unable to govern blood, chronic condition)

Symptoms: Pale gums, lips, and nails due to blood deficiency. Easily bruised. *Tongue*: Pale with white coat. *Pulse*: Soft, weak. *Formula*: Gui Pi Tang (#1 formula for purpura-bruising).

Black teeth (black from inside of teeth, not due to coffee, etc.)

Xue stage heat in the lower Jiao

Symptoms: High fever, delirium, semi-conscious, coma, convulsions. Irritability. Shrivelling and dry lips. *Tongue*: Red with very dry coat, shrunken. *Pulse*: Extremely rapid. *Causes*: Heat has damaged yin and Jin/Ye, stomach ch'i damaged (shrunken mouth). Kidney unable to nourish teeth, turning them black, the colour of the kidneys. *Formula*: Salty, cold, sweet and moist herbs. Fu Mai Tang. Pa Ting Fen Zhu Tang.

Stiffness of neck

Wind cold

Symptoms: More chills than fever, etc. *Tongue*: White slippery coat (slightly greasy). *Pulse*: Floating and tense. *Formula*: Ge Gen Tang.

Wind cold damp (a Bi syndrome such as arthritis)

Symptoms: Heavy sensation in the head, headache, aching joints, fever/chills sometimes. *Tongue*: Greasy coat. *Pulse*: Floating and slippery. *Formula*: Ge Gen Tang + Ch'iang Huo, Jian Huang and/or Sang Zhi.

Xue Stage Heat

Symptoms: High fever, stiffness of head. Irritability, delirium. Possibly associated with convulsions, muscle spasms. 'Extreme heat leads to liver wind'. *Formula*: Ling Yang Ge Gen Tang.

Goitre (enlargement of thyroid gland)

Accumulation of phlegm and ch'i stagnation

Symptoms: Swelling of thyroid, which is soft without pain. Sense of obstruction in throat. Chest constriction and hypochondriac distending pain. Irritability. *Tongue*: Greasy white coat. *Pulse*: Wiry and slippery.

Causes: Stress leads to ch'i stagnation leading to impairment of body fluid metabolism, leading to phlegm congealing in throat. *Formula*: Ban Xia Huo Po Tang +Hai Zao and Kun Bu.

Ch'i and blood stagnation

Symptoms: Tumours or cancer of the thyroid gland developing from accumulation of phlegm and ch'i stagnation (see above). Swelling is harder than simple phlegm and ch'i stagnation. More defined pain and sense of obstruction affecting ability to breathe and/or swallow. Chest constriction and hypochondriac distending pain. Irritability. *Tongue*: Dark purple. *Pulse*: Deep and choppy. *Causes*: Prolonged ch'i stagnation with phlegm leads to hardening of the phlegm leading to tumour formation. *Formula*: Ban Xia Huo Po Tang + blood activators such as E Zhu, San Lin, Dan Shen, Ru Xiang, Mo Ya and anti-cancer herbs.

Yin Xu of the heart and liver

Symptoms: Typical hyperthyroidism, swollen thyroid, though not hard. Palpitations, insomnia, nervous, trembling. Easily sweats, shortness of breath, irritability, dizziness/vertigo. Dry eyes, hot flushes, night sweats. Nocturnal emissions, premature ejaculation. Irregular menstruation. *Tongue*: Red with scanty coat. *Pulse*: Wiry and rapid, or thready and rapid. *Treatment*: Tonify yin and clear fire. *Formulas*: Suan Zao Ren Tang. Zhi Bai Di Huang. Tian Wang Bu Xing Tang. Yi Guan Jiang.

Oedema of the extremities

Accumulation of heat and damp ('Heat Bi')

Symptoms: Oedema in small joints. Acute achy swollen arthritis. Combined with fever, thirst and irritability. *Tongue*: Red body with yellow greasy coat. *Pulse*: Slippery and rapid. *Formula*: Bai Hu Tang + Gui Zhi and Cang Zhu.

Accumulation of cold and damp ('Cold Bi')

Symptoms: Cold, achy arthritis with oedema. *Tongue*: Greasy white coat. *Pulse*: Slow. *Formula*: Wu Tou Tang.

Ch'i stagnation

Symptoms: Pitting oedema. Chest constriction and hypochondriac distending pain. *Tongue*: Pale with white coating. *Pulse*: Wiry. *Causes*: Because this a channel pathology, the cause is often an external pathogen associated with Wind. *Treatment*: Harmonise Ying and Wei ch'i. *Formula*: Xiang Su San. Xiang Fu activates ch'i. Su Ye expels wind.

Ch'i and blood stagnation (post-stroke sequelae, paralysis, hemiplegia)

Symptoms: Oedema (mostly lower extremities), weakness, numbness. Colour of the skin at affected site is purple. *Tongue*: Pale with purple spots. *Pulse*: Wiry, choppy. *Causes*: Phlegm remaining in channels after stroke. *Formula*: Huang Ch'i Gui Zhi Tang.

Stiffness of the extremities

Wind cold and damp

Symptoms: Cold, achy arthritis. *Tongue*: Greasy white coat. *Pulse*: Slow. *Formula*: Gui Zhi Tang, Ge Gen Tang.

Heat and phlegm

Symptoms: High fever, stiffness of extremities. Irritability, delirium. Possibly associated with convulsions, muscle spasms. 'Extreme heat leads to liver wind'. *Formula*: Ling Yang Ge Gen Tang.

Flaccid paralysis of extremities 'Wei syndrome' (usually without pain)

Body Damaged by lung Heat

Symptoms: Follows febrile disease. Usually lower extremities. Low-grade fever and yin impairment. *Tongue*: Red with yellow or scanty coat. *Treatment*: Tonify yin and Jin Ye. *Formula*: Shao Shen Mail Men Dong Tang + San Miao San. Ch'ing Zao Jie Fei Tang. *Acupuncture points*: Yang Ming points. Stomach channel for legs, LI for arms.

Ch'i deficiency of the spleen/stomach

Symptoms: Weakness (not paralysis) of limbs, normal movement, but very weak. Bloating, indigestion, loose stool, aversion to cold, pale complexion. *Tongue*: Pale. *Pulse*: Thready and weak. Prevalent during post-illness recovery period. *Formula*: Bu Zhong Yi Ch'i Tang.

Deficiency of liver and kidney

Symptoms: Old age, or following illness. Hypersensitivity of extremities leading to weakness leading to paralysis. Sore lower back, dysmennorrhea, premature ejaculation. Dizziness, vertigo, fatigue. *Tongue*: Pale. *Pulse*: Deep, thready, weak. Jing deficiency, sometimes combined with ch'i or yin Xu. *Treatment*: Tonifiy Jing and liver (for tendons). *Formula*: Zuo Gui Yin. You Gin Gui Yin. Da Bu Yin Wan.

Blood stagnation

Symptoms: Weakness leading to numbness. Possible spasm leading to paralysis. Tongue: Purple. *Pulse*: Choppy, thready. *Causes*: Poststroke sequelae or tissue trauma. Phlegm remains in channels after stroke. *Treatment*: Promote blood circulation. *Formula*: Tao Hong Si Wu Tang.

Varicoses of the lower extremities

Accumulation of heat and damp (acute condition)

Symptoms: Varicose veins are combined with red, swollen legs. Veins are hot and burning. Fever, bitter taste in the mouth, irregular bowel movements. *Tongue*: Red with yellow greasy coating. *Pulse*: Wiry/rapid. *Causes*: Excessive alcohol intake, damp and heat producing foods. *Treatment*: Clear heat, drain damp. *Formula*: San Miao San. *Points*: Local points that are inserted around the varicose veins, like Hua Toe Jia Jie. Points around the spine. Needles are considered more effective than herbs for this sort of varicose condition.

Accumulation of cold and damp (chronic condition)

Symptoms: Varicose veins are combined with heavy extremities and distension. Blue or purple veins, chronic. Copious urine, loose stools. *Tongue*: White, greasy coat. *Pulse*: Soft. *Causes*: Standing up too much, working environment. *Treatment*: Remove cold and damp. *Formula*: Ji Ming San.

Ch'i deficiency and blood stagnation

Symptoms: Chronic physical weakness or ch'i deficiency. Chronically carrying heavy things and/or standing for a long time. Purple veins. Not as 'big' as in damp/cold accumulation. Achy, but not distended. Fatigue, shortness of breath, pale complexion. *Tongue*: Pale. *Pulse*: Weak. *Treatment*: Harmonise Ying, tonify ch'i, activate blood. *Formula*: Bu Yang Huang Wu Tang.

Feet pain

Liver and kidney deficiency (old age, Jing Xu)

Symptoms: Pain in heel (key symptom). No skin change. Pain worsened by walking or fatigue. Tinnitus, sore back. *Formula*: Hu Jian Wan (patent formula).

Accumulation of cold and damp

Symptoms: Achy joints exasperated by cold and damp. *Tongue*: White coat. *Pulse*: Soft. *Formula*: Dang Gui Si Ni Tang.

Back pain

Accumulation of cold and damp

Symptoms: Pain which can radiate to neck. Back feels heavy, stiff. Symptoms aggravated by cold damp weather. *Formula*: Ch'iang Huo Ji Sheng Tang.

Ch'i and blood stagnation due to recent trauma (acute)

Symptoms: Sudden onset of pain. Limited range of motion, acute symptoms. *Pulse*: Tense. Could develop into chronic pain. *Formula*: Yuen Lian Bai Yao. Huo Lou Xiao Ling Dan.

Ch'i and blood stagnation due to past trauma (chronic)

Symptoms: Dull aching on/off, numbness aggravated by rest (deficiency beneath). *Tongue*: Purple. *Pulse*: Thready and/or choppy. *Treatment*:

Tonify and activate ch'i and blood. *Formula*: Du Huo Ji Sheng Wan + Tao Ren and Hong Hua.

Weakness of the lower back and knees

Kidney/liver deficiency formulas are Zuo Gui Wan, Rou Gui Wan, Bao Wei Di Huang Want, Liu Wei Di Huang Wan.

Jing deficiency

Symptoms: Infertility, tinnitus, vertigo, sore back, premature ejaculation, amenorrhea, grey hair, premature ageing. *Formulas*. Kidney/liver formulas plus Zi He Che, Lu Rong.

Yin deficiency

Symptoms: Emaciation, tidal fever, heat signs, five centre heat. *Formulas*: Kidney/liver formulas plus Huang Bai, Zhi Mu.

Yang deficiency

Symptoms: Cold signs such as cold hands and feet. *Formulas*: Kidney/liver tonic formulas plus Fu Zi, Ba Ji Tian, Bu Gu Zi.

Ch'i deficiency

Symptoms: Weakness of the lower gates (urethra, colon, etc) incontinence, premature ejaculation, urination problems. *Formulas*: Kidney/liver tonic formulas plus astringent herbs such as Sang Pian Xiao, Yi Zhi Ren, Wu Wei Zi, Fu Peng Zi.

Chest pain (often connected to the heart)

Heart ch'i deficiency

Symptoms: Mild pain. Neurosis, heart condition. Dull achy chest pain on one or both sides. Chest congestion, palpitations. Spontaneous sweating, fatigue. *Tongue*: Pale. *Pulse*: Weak and thready. *Treatment*: Tonify heart ch'i. *Formula*: Bao Yuan Wan.

Cold accumulation (yang deficiency) painful

Symptoms: Coronary heart disease. Chest pain, usually on the left side which could radiate to the right, back shoulder, and arm. Pale complexion, spontaneous sweating, cold extremities. *Tongue*: Pale, swollen, teeth marks. *Pulse*: Deep, slow, knotty and intermittent. *Treatment*: Tonify heart yang, promote circulation of blood. *Formula*: Gua Luo Xie Bai. Bai Jiu Tang.

Heart blood stagnation (still a form of yang Xu)

Symptoms: Typical angina pectoris. Intense pain that can make the patient lose consciousness. Spontaneous cold sweating, fear, fatigue. *Tongue*: Pale purple. *Pulse*: Deep, thready, choppy, knotty, intermittent. *Herb*: Dan Shen for chest pain. *Formula*: Xue Fu Zhu Yu Tang. Ge Xian Zhu Yu Tang.

Mass formation in the abdomen

Ch'i and Xue stagnation

Symptoms: Enlargement of the liver and spleen. Abdominal mass begins soft, but becomes harder as time goes by. Distension, emaciation, fatigue. Dark, dull facial complexion. Poor appetite, dry skin. *Tongue*: Purple spots. *Pulse*: Wiry, tense. Cancerous tumours tend to be more blood stagnation than ch'i stagnation. *Treatment*: Activate blood, yin deficiency unimportant now. *Formula*: Ge Xian Zhu Yu Tang + Shi Xiao San.

Phlegm stagnation

Symptoms: Abdominal mass, no pain, yet distended and uncomfortable. Mass is movable and soft, but patient dislikes touch. *Tongue*: Pale. *Pulse*: Soft and slippery. *Formula*: Ban He Wan. Er Chan Tang.

Zhong ch'i Xu (sinking, or organ prolapsed)

Symptoms: Pulling down, or bearing down sensation. Ch'i deficiency symptoms. *Formula*: Bu Zhong Yi Ch'i Tang.

Tenesmus

Accumulation of damp, heat, and toxic heat

Symptoms: Tenesmus, diarrhoea, abdominal pain, blood and mucus in stool. Pus and burning sensation in anus, possible fever. Yellow scanty urine. *Tongue*: Red with yellow coat. *Pulse*: Slippery and rapid. *Formula*: Dan Gui Xhao Yao Tang.

Constipation

Yang Ming Heat (Yang Ming Fu LI)

Symptoms: Fever, constipation, abdominal discomfort, dislikes palpation. Feels mass in abdomen. *Pulse*: Deep, strong and slow due to stagnation. *Treatment*: Purge heat and stagnation. *Formula*: Da Ching Ch'i Tang.

Ch'i stagnation

Symptoms: Constipation. Depression, easily angered, chest congestion discomfort in hypochondrium, distension and discomfort in breast, water retention (due to digestive problems, secondary to the stagnation). *Formula*: Chai Hu Su Gan Tang + lubricative herbs such as Tao Ren or Huo Ma Ren.

Ch'i deficiency

Symptoms: Constipation, sometimes loose. Extreme fatigue especially after a bowel movement. Weak voice. Possible rectal prolapse. *Tongue*: Pale with white coat. *Pulse*: Weak. *Formula*: Bu Zhong Yi Ch'i Tang.

Blood and yin Xu

Symptoms: Chronic, old age patients. Constipation, emaciation, dry skin. palpitations, pale complexion. *Tongue*: Pale, red or narrow. *Pulse*: Thready and rapid. *Herbs*: Dang Gui, Sheng Di Huang, Rou Cong Ren. *Formula*: Wu Ren Wan. Sheng Ye Cheng Ch'i Tang.

Incontinence of faeces (all serious conditions)

Accumulation of heat and toxins

Symptoms: Xue level heat and toxin. High fever, delirium. Semiconsciousness, coma, excess diarrhoea with pus and blood. *Tongue*: Red with yellow coat. *Pulse*: Rapid. *Treatment*: Clear blood level heat *Formula*: Xi Jiao Di Huang Tang.

Spleen, kidney yang Xu

Symptoms: Chronic diarrhoea/dysentery. Diarrhoea with mucus, incontinence of faeces. Fatigue, cold, low back pain. *Tongue*: Pale. *Pulse*: Deep, thready, weak. *Formula*: Zheng Ren Yang Zhong Tang.

Spleen ch'i sinking (extreme weak condition)

Symptoms: Incontinence of faeces, rectal prolapse, tired, disorientated. *Tongue*: Pale. *Pulse*: Feeble. *Formula*: Shen Fu Tang.

Incontinence of urine

Kidney ch'i deficiency

(Common among the elderly and those recovering from serious illness)

Symptoms: Frequent urination and incontinence, mostly in the evening. Kidney ch'i and/or yang Xu symptoms. *Tongue*: Pale. *Pulse*: Deep, weak especially in the kidney positions.

Cloudy urination

Accumulation of damp heat (excess turbid damp, acute)

Symptoms: Cloudy urine with white or yellow urine. Frequent, burning, urgent, painful urination. Fever, thirst. *Tongue*: Red with yellow coat. *Pulse*: Wiry and thready. *Formula*: Ba Zheng San + Shi Chang Pu. Pi Xie Feng Ch'ing Yin.

Kidney yin or yang deficiency

(Deficiency syndrome in which the essence leaks out with the urine)

Symptoms: Chronic cloudy urine. Yin Xu symptoms: Scanty yellow urine. *Tongue*: Red. *Pulse*: Thready and rapid. Yang Xu symptoms: Copious clear urine. *Tongue*: Pale. *Pulse*: Deep and weak. Kidneys are unable to govern the essence in the kidneys. *Treatment*: Tonify kidneys. Astringent essence formulas. For kidney yin Xu – Zhi Bai Di Huang Wan + Pi Xia, Fu Pen Zi, Wu Wei Zi, Tu Si Zi (all astringents). For kidney yang Xu – You Gui Yin or Wan + Pi Xia, Fu Pen Zi, Wu Wei Zi, Tu Si Zi (all astringents).

Frequent urination in evening (often found in the elderly)

Kidney Ch'i Xu or Kidney Yang Xu. *Formulas*: Sang Piao Xie San + You Gui Wan. For prostate problems: Kai Kit Wan.

Oliguria, or difficult urination

Damp heat

Symptoms: Cloudy yellow urine. Frequent, burning, urgent, painful urination, incontinence. *Formula*: Ba Zheng San + Shi Chang Pu. Pi Xie Feng Ch'ing Yin.

Lung ch'i stagnation (lungs unable to descend the water)

Symptoms: Cough, chest congestion, constipation. *Tongue*: Red. *Pulse*: Soft and rapid. *Formula*: Ch'ing Feng Wan.

Zhong Ch'i Xu (spleen ch'i sinking)

Symptoms: Urination lacking strength, sluggish stream. Fatigue, bearing down sense. Urine frequent but small amounts. Loose stool. *Tongue*: Pale. *Pulse*: Thready and weak. *Formula*: Bu Zhong Yi Ch'i Tang.

Kidney ch'i Xu

Symptoms: Difficult urination, sluggish stream, incontinence. Frequent urination. Kidney problems in Western medicine. *Treatment*: Tonify kidney. *Formula*: Ba Wei Di Huang Wan.

Stagnation of urinary tract (common after abdominal surgery or trauma)

Symptoms: Sluggish, difficult urination. Abdominal distension of pain. *Tongue*: Purple, possibly with raised purple bumps. *Pulse*: Choppy. *Formula*: Chong Xian San.

Seminal fluid in urine

Accumulation of damp heat

This applies largely to what the Western world would call sexually transmitted diseases (STDs).

Symptoms: Frequent, cloudy, sluggish, burning urine. Sticky white discharge following urination. Bitter taste in mouth. Thirst, chest congestion, sluggish bowels. *Tongue*: Red with yellow greasy coat. *Pulse*: Soft and rapid (if more damp), or slippery and rapid (if more heat). *Treatment*: Dry damp, clear heat. *Formula*: Pi Xie Feng Ch'ing Yin.

Kidney yin Xu with empty heat

Symptoms: Frequent, cloudy, burning urine. White or red discharge after urination. Dizziness, vertigo, insomnia, restlessness. Tidal fever, yin Xu symptoms. *Tongue*: Red with dry coat. *Pulse*: Thready and rapid. *Treatment*: Tonify yin and Jing. *Formula*: Shi Bai Di Huang Wan + astringents such as Tu Si Zi, Jing Yin Zi, Wu Wei Zi.

Kidney ch'i or yang Xu (Very weak people, not an STD)

Symptoms: Frequent, copious, clear urine. seminal fluid discharge following urination. Premature ejaculation, impotence, nocturnal emissions. *Tongue*: Pale. *Pulse*: Deep and weak. *Formula*: You Gui Wan and astringents.

Blood in seminal fluid

Yin deficiency with intense empty heat

Symptoms: Blood in ejaculate. Distension and pain in testes or penis. Burning sensation in urinary tract. Emaciation. Thirst, irritability. *Tongue*: Red with scanty coat. *Pulse*: thready and rapid. *Treatment*: Tonify yin, clear fire, harmonise blood, stop the bleeding. *Formula*: Zhi Bai Di Huang Wan or Da Bu yin Wen + E Jiao or bleeding.

Damp heat accumulation (STD)

Symptoms: Blood in ejaculate. Frequent painful urination. Pain, burning, itching in urinary tract. Spasms of pain in testicles. Blood in urine. *Tongue*: Greasy yellow coat. *Pulse*: Slippery, wiry, rapid. *Formula*: Bai Zhen San + Da Ch'ing Ye, Huang Ch'in, Huang Bai, Zhi Zi, Bai Bu.

Thin and scanty ejaculate (Western differentiation: low sperm count)

Kidney ch'i deficiency, or kidney yang deficiency

Symptoms: Infertility, very chronic fatigue, pale complexion, sore or weak lower back, senility, hair loss and loose teeth, hearing loss, frequent urination – especially in evening. *Tongue*: Pale. *Pulse*: Weak in kidney position. *Treatment*: Tonify kidney ch'i, yang, and essence. *Formula*: You Gui Wan.

Cold stagnation (yang deficiency condition)

Symptoms: Scanty semen. Infertility, very chronic fatigue, pale complexion, sore or weak lower back, senility, hair loss and loose teeth, hearing loss, frequent urination – especially in evening. Cold extremities, testicles. *Formula*: You Gui Wan + Fu Zi, Ba Ji Tian, Suo Yang.

Inability to ejaculate during intercourse

Yin deficiency with empty heat

Symptoms: Distension in scrotum. Possible nocturnal emissions, irritability, scanty urine, constipation, thirst. *Tongue*: Red. *Pulse*: Thready and rapid. *Treatment*: Tonify yin to move stagnation. *Formula*: Zhi Bai Di Huang Wan + Mu Tong, Wang Bu Liu Xin.

Blood stagnation due to chronic stress

Ch'i stagnation leading to blood stagnation. Liver stagnates ch'i, and the channel passes through the gonads. *Symptoms*: Easily angered, chest congestion. Varicose of scrotum (vericoseal). *Tongue*: Purple. *Pulse*: Deep and choppy. *Formula*: Xu Fu Zhu Yu Tang + Jiu Zi, Ch'i Cuang Zi.

Premature ejaculation

Kidney ch'i or yang Xu

Symptoms: Impotence, sore back, hair loss, loose teeth, senility. *Tongue*: Pale. *Pulse*: Weak at kidney point. *Formula*: You Gui Wan, Ba Wei Di Huang Wan.

Deficiency of heart and spleen

Symptoms: Neurosis (if there's a psychological component). Impotence, emaciation, fatigue, pale complexion. Palpitations, insomnia, forgetfulness. indigestion. *Tongue*: Pale. *Pulse*: Weak. *Formula*: Gui Pi Tang.

Nocturnal emissions (more heat)/ Spermatorrhea (more cold)

Heart and spleen deficiency

Symptoms: Impotence, emaciation, fatigue, pale complexion. Palpitations, insomnia, forgetfulness, indigestion. *Tongue*: Pink or red. *Pulse*: Weak or thready. *Treatment*: Clear heat, subdue fire and calm Shen. Astringent essence. *Formula*: Tian Wan Bu Xing Tang + Bai Shao, E Jiao.

Liver fire (nocturnal emissions)

Symptoms: Bitter taste in mouth. Dark urine. Easily angered. *Pulse*: Wiry. *Formula*: Long Dan Xie Gan Tang.

Kidney ch'i Xu (Spermatorrhea)

Symptoms: Tinnitus, dizziness, fatigue, sore or weak lower back. *Formula*: You Gui Wan + astringent herbs.

Accumulation of damp heat

Symptoms: Irritability, fever, itching. Burning sensation in lower abdomen or testicles. Scanty yellow urine. *Tongue*: Yellow, greasy coat. *Pulse*: Wiry, slippery. *Formula*: Long Dan Xie Gan Tang + Ba Zhen Tang.

Impotence

Kidney yang Xu

Symptoms: Cold testes, soreness and weakness in the lower back and knees. Poor memory, hearing and hair loss, loose teeth, aversion to cold and cold extremities. Ch'i Xu symptoms. *Tongue*: Pale and swollen with teeth marks. *Pulse*: Deep thready, weak, especially in kidney positions. *Causes*: Age, too much sexual activity, constitutional weakness. *Treatment*: Warm and stimulate kidney yang. *Formula*: You Gui Yin or Wan.

Heart/spleen deficiency (psychogenic, in Western terms)

Symptoms: Palpitations, shortness of breath, emaciation, insomnia, restlessness, vivid dreams, fatigue, indigestion, bloating, loose stools. *Tongue*: Pale. *Pulse*: Thready. *Causes*: Thinking or worrying too much creates the spleen Zi deficiency which leads to ch'i and blood deficiency, which creates a heart blood deficiency, leading to various neuroses. Plus, the ch'i and blood can't support the essence, which leads to impotence. *Treatment*: Tonify heart and spleen. *Formula*: Gui Pi Tang + kidney tonic herbs which will warm the spleen, such as Bu Gu Zi, Ba Ji Tian, Xian Ma.

Impotence due to fear

Symptoms: Frustration, easily panicked, insomnia, vivid dreams and nightmares, erection up until intercourse begins. Tongue and pulse can be normal. *Treatment*: Calm Shen. *Formula*: Ting Zhi Wan + Shi Chang Pu, Ren Shen, Yuan Zhi.

Persistent erection

Damp heat in liver (lasts days or even months)

Symptoms: Penis is dark purple, distended pain, difficult urination, scanty dark yellow urine, fear, bitter taste in mouth, thirst, constipation. *Tongue*: Red with yellow coat. *Pulse*: Wiry, slippery, rapid. *Treatment*: Clear heat, dry damp. *Formula*: Long Dan Xie Gan Tang.

Yin Xu with intense empty heat

Symptoms: Emaciation, high sex drive, distension and pain, though slight compared to damp heat in liver. Sometimes scanty urine. Flushed, nervousness, hyperactive, easily anxious. *Tongue*: Red and narrow, scanty coat. *Pulse*: Thready and rapid. *Treatment*: Tonify yin, clear heat. *Formula*: Zhi Bai Di Huang Wan.

Coldness in the external genitalia (both men and women)

Kidney yang Xu with interior cold or Ming Men Xu

Symptoms: Impotence, premature ejaculation (male). Low sexual desire (female). *Tongue*: Pale with teeth marks. *Pulse*: Deep, slow and weak. *Formula*: Ba Hui Di Huang Wan + Lu Rong and Wu Zhu Yu.

Flaccid retraction of the penis

Cold stagnation

Symptoms: Cold extremities and body, purple lips, severe muscle aches and abdominal cramping, maybe diarrhoea. *Tongue*: Normal. *Pulse*: Deep, slow and weak, or deep, slow and tense. *Causes*: Constitutional yang Xu + pathogenic cold or just pathogenic cold in the liver channel leading to cold stagnation which blocks ch'i and blood in the channels that pass through the genital area. *Treatment*: Warm and remove cold stagnation. *Formula*: Wu Zhu Yu Tang or Dang Gui Si Ni Tang.

Yang collapse

(This is a critical condition, the liver is dying.) *Symptoms*: Spontaneous cold sweating. Semi-consciousness or unconsciousness. *Treatment*: Obviously the penile retraction will be secondary to the more immediate need to rescue and restore the yang before the patient expires. *Formula*: Gui Yang Tang.

Itching and burning in the genitalia

Damp heat in the liver channel

Symptoms: Burning, difficult, dark, painful and frequent urination. Cloudy urine, fever thirst. *Tongue*: Yellow, greasy. *Pulse*: Slippery, wiry, rapid. *Treatment*: Clear damp, clear heat. *Formula*: Long Dan Xie Gan Tang.

Heat and fire accumulation

Symptoms: Burning and heat in genitals, fever, mouth ulcers, thirst, more heat symptoms. *Tongue*: Red, especially the tip. *Pulse*: Rapid. *Treatment*: Clear heat, clear fire. *Formula*: Da Ch'i San.

Blood stagnation

Symptoms: Severe, excruciating pain, burning in urinary tract. Kidney, or urinary tract stones, bloody urine, cloudy urine. Pain referred to the abdomen or lower back. *Tongue*: Purple spots. *Pulse*: Deep and choppy. *Formula*: Tao Hong Si Wu Tang + Ba Zhen San.

Light menstrual flow

Ch'i and blood Xu

Symptoms: Light flow, delayed cycle, abdominal aching, fatigue, dizziness. *Tongue*: Pale. *Pulse*: Thready. Anaemia. Heavy flow possible in the case of ch'i Xu with no blood Xu. *Formula*: Ba Zhen Tang.

Accumulation of phlegm damp

Symptoms: Light flow, obese patient, irregular cycles, heavy sensation in body. *Tongue*: Swollen tongue body with greasy coat. *Pulse*: Soft and slippery. *Formula*: Chuang Gui Er Chen Tang.

Dark purple or thick menstrual flow

Ch'i and blood stagnation

Symptoms: Dark purple flow with clots, severe abdominal pain, severe pre-menstrual syndrome symptoms. *Tongue*: Purple. *Pulse*: Choppy. *Formula*: Tao He Cheng Ch'i Tang.

Heat and blood stagnation

Symptoms: Thick, dark, clotty flow. Severe abdominal pain, fever, mental symptoms. *Formula*: Tao He Si Wu Tang.

Cold stagnation leading to blood stagnation

Symptoms: Thick, dark, clotty, flow. Severe abdominal pain, fever, mental symptoms. Lower back cold, patient prefers warmth. *Tongue*: White coat. *Pulse*: Deep and tense. *Formula*: Wen Jing Tang.

Thick menstrual flow

Ch'i and blood stagnation

Symptoms: Dark purple flow with clots, severe abdominal pain, severe pre-menstrual syndrome symptoms. *Tongue*: Purple. *Pulse*: Choppy. *Formula*: Tao He Cheng Ch'i Tang.

Heat and blood stagnation

Symptoms: Thick, dark, clotty flow. Severe abdominal pain, fever, mental symptoms. *Formula*: Tao He Si Wu Tang.

Cold stagnation leading to blood stagnation

Symptoms: Thick, dark, clotty flow. Severe abdominal pain, fever, mental symptoms. Lower back cold, patient prefers warmth. *Tongue*: White coat. *Pulse*: Deep and tense. *Formula*: Wen Jing Tang.

Amenorrhea (lack of period)

Kidney ch'i deficiency

Symptoms: Congenital kidney ch'i deficiency (primary amenorrhea). No period as of the 15th birthday. Emaciation, lower back pain, fatigue, slow development. *Pulse*: Weak. *Tongue*: Pale. *Treatment*: Tonify kidney.

Ch'i and blood deficiency

Symptoms: Usually found after an illness or *post partum*. No pain, no period. Palpitations. Fatigue, weakness. *Pulse*: Weak. *Treatment*: Tonify ch'i and blood. *Formula*: Ba Zhen Tang.

Ch'i and blood stagnation

Symptoms: Amenorrhea following traumatic injury or stress. Lots of distension and pain. Fatigue, depression, anger. *Tongue*: Varies. *Pulse*: Deep and wiry.

Damp and phlegm accumulation

Symptoms: Menopausal symptoms. Delayed cycle, quantity of flow is light. Amenorrhea, weight gain, water retention. *Tongue*: Pale with white greasy coat. *Pulse*: Soft and slippery.

Metohrragia (heavy flow)

Ch'i and blood deficiency

Symptoms: Heavy quantity, thin quality and light colour. *Treatment*: Tonify ch'i and blood. *Formula*: Ba Zhen Tang.

Heat in blood

Symptoms: Dark red flow

Blood stagnation

Symptoms: Irregular flow, spotting, dark purple colour clots, pain in abdomen, which gets better after the onset of the flow. *Tongue*: Purple. *Pulse*: Deep and choppy, or wiry and slippery.

Irregular menstrual cycle

Liver ch'i stagnation

Accounts for most cases, though a few are caused by kidney ch'i deficiency. *Formula*: Xiao Yao San.

Fever during menstruation

Liver ch'i stagnation with liver fire (most common)

Symptoms: Fever alternating with chills, more often before period, sometimes during. Early or irregular cycle, irritation, dizziness. Thirst, dry mouth. *Tongue*: Red with yellow coat. *Pulse*: Wiry and rapid.

Yin deficiency fever

Symptoms: Fever following illness of *post partum*. This fever tends to happen before or during the period. Emaciation, irritability, dry mouth, thirst. *Tongue*: Red and thin. *Pulse*: Thready and rapid.

Wind cold

Symptoms: Chong and Ren channels are weak just prior to menses. Tai Yang syndrome. *Formula*: Gui Pi Tang even if there's no sweating. Xiao Chai Hu Tang if fever is also associated with chills.

Blood stagnation before or during period

Symptoms: Abdominal pain, dark complexion. Flow is purple with clots. *Formula*: Xue Fu Zhu Yu Tang.

Ch'i deficiency or ch'i and blood deficiency fever

Symptoms: Fever before or during the period. Light colour and thin quality, scanty quantity. *Tongue*: Pale. *Pulse*: Weak. *Formula*: Bu Zhong Yi Ch'i Tang.

8

COMMONLY ASKED QUESTIONS

We look at it, and we do not see it, and we name it 'the Equable.'
We listen to it, and we do not hear it, and we name it 'the
Inaudible'. We try to grasp it, and do not get hold of it, and we
name it 'the Subtle'.With these three qualities, it cannot be made
the subject of description; and hence we blend them together and
obtain The One.

Tao Ti Ching

What is traditional Chinese medicine?

A method of restoring energy balance (ch'i) to promote healing and functioning through inserting needles at precise points on the body. Heat is often applied over acupuncture point ('moxibustion') to strengthen (ch'i).

How does it work?

Meridians, channels of energy, run like energy currents throughout the body. When blockage in one part of a channel occurs, it impedes the flow in others. Acupuncture removes the blockage and revives the usual flow through the meridians, restoring ch'i and helping the body's internal organs with imbalances.

Acupuncture's scientific rationale is that inserting needles at acupuncture points stimulates the nervous system, releasing chemicals which either alleviate pain or affect the body's internal regulating system.

How can acupuncture help?

It can impact positively health and wellness, treatment of various medical conditions and prevention of illness. Most often associated with pain control, acupuncture is also used for many medical disorders – either by itself, or in support of other medical treatment.

Acupuncture is acknowledged by the World Health Organisation for treatment of numerous medical conditions including: digestive disorders; respiratory ailments; neurological and muscular maladies; and urinary, menstrual and reproductive problems. It is especially helpful with physical difficulties caused by tension and stress.

Are there side-effects?

Infrequently. At times, after acupuncture treatment, an individual's symptoms can intensify for a short time. Most often, a period of relaxation is experienced.

Do the needles hurt?

Most people feel only minimal pain; some feel no pain at all. After the needles have been inserted, one may feel a sensation of heaviness or tingling.

Is there a risk of infection?

Because needles are disposable, or are sterilised as surgical instruments are, there is no risk of infection.

How many treatments are needed?

This varies with the individual and is dependent on whether the patient has an acute condition, an enduring or difficult problem, or is treated for health maintenance. The number of treatments vary from as many as one or two a week for several months to as few as four a year.

Is it really effective?

For 2,000 years it has been successfully used to treat more people than are treated with all other health methods combined. Acupuncture is currently widely practised in countries around the world, and is increasingly used in the US. The United Nations supports its use.

Does health insurance cover acupuncture?

Coverage of acupuncture is rapidly changing, and is dependent on each insurance company's policy. State law requires California-based insurance providers to offer acupuncture, a modality of treatment, as part of their coverage. Please check with your insurance company and encourage them to include coverage of acupuncture treatment.

What is herbal medicine?

Herbal medicine is an integral part of healing in Chinese medicine, as it is in many other cultures. A herbalist works to match the therapeutic characteristics and nature of herbs to formulate a prescription that will meet the patient's individual needs.

What is Tai Ch'i?

Once of the principal branches of Chinese martial arts internal style, Tai Ch'i draws from martial arts, Taoist philosophy, and medicine. It is composed of slow and graceful fluid movements that keep the body in motion and the mind tranquil. Tai Ch'i is an exercise through which we connect with the essence of our energy, learn to harness it, and let it flow naturally – harmonising that energy.

Tai Ch'i provides strength and flexibility to the body, tranquillity and serenity to the mind, and brings a sense of well-being to the practitioner. It rejuvenates and revitalises.

What is Ch'i Kung?

A practice for the cultivation of ch'i, Ch'i Kung is a way to harness internal energy for the enhancement of energy flow in the body. It is a meditative process that is often used in China for patients with chronic and severe illness.

Can acupuncture help cancer?

The latest issue of the *Chinese Medical Journal*, the only English-language medical journal in China, published by the Chinese Medical Association, has run two articles about the treatment of cancer with traditional Chinese medicine. Adapted excerpts follow:

According to the theories of traditional Chinese medicine, cancer is the result of the long-term action of cancer-producing elements under a physical condition termed 'internal insufficiency'. Some chronic inflammatory changes may cause epithelial cells to proliferate and turn malignant. Thus, it's very important for doctors of traditional Chinese medicine to treat injuries or other alterations of any organ or tissue before such changes result in impairment or loss of function which might then result in the development of cancerous cells.

Some Chinese herbs possess the medicinal properties that may help prevent cancer cells from growing, reduce the disturbance of the body's internal environment and inhibit the development of cancer-inducing injuries.

Animal experiments, for instance, reveal that Chinese herbs such as Chinese angelica (Angelica sinesis or Dang Gui in Chinese) and Chinese magnoliavine (Schizandra sinensis, or Wuweizi in Chinese) can inhibit liver cancer induced by aflatoxin, a group of toxic compounds produced by a type of fungus.

Research is going on in areas where there are high percentages of throat cancer. The focus of the studies is a herbal decoction, Liuwei Dihuang Tang, which is effective in interrupting severely abnormal formation of tissue in the throat. Laboratory tests have demonstrated that ginsenoside (Rb2), the main component of Chinese ginseng, can destroy Melanoma B16, cells that cause skin cancer.

Cancer treatment

The key feature of traditional Chinese medicine is the concept that the human body is a whole and that its parts cannot be treated separately; a symptom may be the result of various other conditions, thus diagnosis should be based on a holistic consideration of all possible causes.

Experiments have shown that the effectiveness of traditional Chinese medicine in treating cancer results mainly from two things. One is the destruction of cancer cells directly, the other is the strengthening of resistance to cancer and the regulation of the function of various body systems.

Comprehensive treatment with traditional Chinese medicine includes complex prescriptions, single medicinal herbs, acupuncture, moxibustion treatment, Ch'i Kung exercise, food therapy, and physical therapy. These different methods of treatment help improve cancer patients' general condition, enhance the functions of the immune system and maintain the internal balance of the body.

Many Chinese herbs and complex prescriptions have been proven to be able to inhibit tumour development by strengthening the patient's immune system. These herbs help increase the cell-mediated immune functions, induce the body to produce more lymphokines, regulate metabolism, and protect the hemopoietic function of bone marrow.

Since traditional Chinese medicine is effective in improving the general condition of patients, restoring the functions of the digestive tract and reducing the occurrence of complications, it has been widely applied to facilitate the recovery of the patient after surgical operation.

The combination of traditional Chinese medicine and Western medicine has been accepted by both doctors and patients, and has become a standard part of cancer prevention and treatment in China.

APPENDIX 1
Acupuncture points

Gravity is the root of lightness; stillness, the ruler of movement.
Tao Ti Ching

The choice of acupuncture points

Acute conditions often respond in 1–4 sessions at intervals of 12–14 hours. Chronic and more difficult conditions may require up to 14 or more sessions at intervals of 3–7 days. As a general rule, if some improvement is not seen by the sixth session, the probability of success becomes less and less with each subsequent non-responding session.

Channel codes used in the Index below are: LU = Lung; LI = large intestine, colon; ST = stomach; SP = spleen–Pancreas; HT = Heart; SI = small intestine; BL = bladder; KI = kidney; PC = pericardium, circulation; sex, heart constrictor; TH = triple heater; GB = gall bladder; LV = liver; GV= governing vessel (Du, dorsal midline); CV = Conception Vessel (Ren, ventral midline).

Z 01-31; Y 01-19; X 01-35; A 01-44; L 01-42 are the 'Strange Points' for head and neck; thorax and abdomen; loin and back; upper limb and lower limb respectively.

NZ01-35; NY01-06; NX01-16; NA01-15; NL01-36 are the 'New Points' for head and neck; abdomen; loin and back; upper limb and lower limb respectively; H are the Hand points.

In this system, ST08 (Tou Wei) is on the temple and BL40 (Wei Zhong) is in the popliteal crease.

These prescriptions are usually in the format of a Primary + Secondary + Tertiary list. The Primary (P) list is the most important. They are regarded as the main points. Points in the Secondary (S) and Tertiary (T) lists are added only if the symptoms dictate. For example, in chronic debilitating diseases, Primary (P) points are: BL43; ST36; X 18. Secondary (S) points are: BL17,20,23; CV06; PC06. If abdominal pain or uterine pathology is present: add CV06; if kidney disease is present: add BL20 (or BL21), etc.

In short prescriptions, the Secondary (S) list could be added as a routine. For example in skin diseases involving malignant pustules, the Primary (P) point is GV12 and the Secondary (S) points (LI04; BL40) could be added routinely.

The laws governing the choice of points should be kept in mind and at least two of them should be fulfilled by the points used. Also consider alternating the choice of points between sessions

The convention *x to y* means a needle penetrating from point *x* to point *y* (for example GB39 to SP06); the convention *x-y* means any or all points between point *x* and point *y* (for example SI10-14).

General conditions

To stimulate immune reaction (antibody production [immunostimulant effect], leucocytosis, phagocytosis in infections or leucopenia) P: LI04,11; GV14; ST36; GB39 to SP06; S: In localised infections add points for the region or organ affected.

Chronic disease (slow convalescence; to improve constitution after debilitating diseases) P: BL43; ST36; X 18; S: BL17,20,23; CV06; PC06.

Weak constitution (fatigue, poor general health, general weakness (as a tonic)) P: CV03,04; ST36; SP06; LI11; BL20,43; S: PC06; SP21; CV12; LI04; HT09; BL10,11; LV03; GV14; GB34,38; X 18.

Fever, hyperthermia P: LI04,11; GV14; S: ST36,44; LU10; Bleed Earpoint 'Apex'; dehydration, thirst: add KI07.

Allergies, hypersensitivities (immunosuppressant effect) P: LI04,11; ST36; GV14; LV03; GB39 to SP06; S: Local allergies: add local and distant points for the region or affected organ; urticaria: add SP10.

Anaemia P: GV14; ST36; BL17; CV04,06; LI11; S: GV04; CV12; BL18,20,22,23; T: PC06; SP06,10; LI04; KI01; GV20.

Anaesthetic emergencies (apnoea, respiratory and cardiac arrest), neonatal asphyxia P: GV26; S: KI01; T: strong stimulation of ear canal.

Muscle cramp, P: Ah Shi points in muscles; forelimb: search forelimb, neck, thoracic muscles. Add main points for cramping region. (Legs, esp. BL23,40,57; GB30,34; Low back especially BL23,25,27,31; GV02,03,04; X 35 [L1-S4]; S: BL40,60; GB30,34; Arms especially GB21; LI11,15; TH05,14; BL11,12,41; X 35 [C1-T6 area]).

Paralysis of peripheral motor nerves, spinal paralysis P: Stimulate nerves (bilaterally), with strong stimulation on affected side. Use local points for the region or affected limb, especially a chain of points over affected nerves. Use Ah Shi points, if present (but they are seldom present). Use the scalp points (on the opposite side) for the motor areas; S: Massage and physiotherapy, if possible. If cerebral anaemia is suspected, add GV26. Consult textbooks for further details.

Disorders of the skin

Neurodermatitis, dermatitis, eczema, urticaria, pruritus P: LI04,11; SP06,10; KI09; ST36; S: LI04,15; GV14; BL13,17,23,25,40; PC07; GB20; ST25; SI03.

Malignant pustules, carbuncles, furuncles, boils, folliculitis (anywhere on the body) P: GV12; S: LI04; BL40.

Abscess, felon, whitlow (nailbed) P: GV10; S: BL40.

Nervous disorders

Epilepsy, during attack P: GV26; KI01; LU11; SI03; BL62; Between attacks P: GV14,20; PC06; HT07; ST36,40; BL15; CV12; Y 29; S: GV06,08,13,24; PC05; HT05; GB20; CV15; SI03; BL62; T: GV01,12,15,16,17; KI06,09; SP01; PC07,08; GV06,17; LI04,11; BL03,05,61,63,64,65; GB09,13,15; ST41,42,45; SI08; TH17; LV02,03; A 01; Z 01.

Convulsions, during attack P: KI01; GV26; Between attacks P: LI04; LV03; SI03; BL20; ST36; S: LU11; LI11; SP01; BL60,63; GB20; LV02; CV04,06,12; GV12,14,21,22.

Hysteria, during attack P: KI01; GV26; Between attacks P: PC06; HT04,07; SP06; GV08; KI01,05: LI04; BL15,22; CV12; GV13,26; ST36,40; SI03; GV14,20.

Unconsciousness, coma P: GV26; KI01; LU11; A 01; S: GV20; PC06,08,09; LV03; HT09; T: LI01,04; ST36; CV06; GV24,25.

Disorders of the neck and thoracic limb

Neck pain, sprain, rheumatism, spasm, arthritis, slipped disc, wry neck and paralysis P: GB20,21,39; BL10,11; GV14,16; SI03,07; X 35 (C2-T4); A 23; Ah Shi; S: BL12,41; SI06,14,15; LI04,11; LU07; TH05,15; BL40,43,60,64,65; SI10,11,16; GB34,36; GV13,18; CV24; TH10,12,16; HT07; LI15; KI01; A 22.

Upper limb pain, sprain, rheumatism, spasm, arthritis P: LI04,11,15; TH05; Ah Shi (neck, back, shoulder area and arm) and local points; S: SI03,06,08; BL11; LI10; T: TH07,14; BL18,40,62; GB34; ST44; NZ23; A 30,32.

Upper limb paralysis P: LI15, LI11 to IIT03; TH09 to TH10; TH05 to PC06; LI04 to PC08 (or LI04 to SI03); S: LI09,10; SI09; A 30; NX04; SI06; GB21; TH03,04.

Shoulder, pain, cramp, rheumatism, stiffness, arthritis, bursitis P: TH14,15; LI11,15,16; BL11; SI09,11; Ah Shi; S: TH10; SI03,10,13; GB21; T: TH03,06,11,13; GV12,14; SI12,14,15; LI04,10; BL13,41,44; A 42.

Shoulder, shoulder muscles and thoracic back pain, spasm, etc. P: LI11,15; SI09,10,11,12,13,14; GB21; TH14; Ah Shi; S: BL11; SI03,08,15; LU02,09; LI02; T: TH03,11,13,15; SI06; LI04; BL12,13,41,42,44; GB20; HT02.

Shoulder and arm muscles: pain, cramp, rheumatism P: LI04,11,15; TH05,14; Ah Shi; S: LI10; TH06,15; GB34; ST36; T: LI07,16; TH10,11,13; SI11.

Elbow pain, sprain, arthritis, rheumatism P: Ah Shi; LI11 to HT03; LI12; LU05; TH05; S: LI04,10; GB34; SI04; T: LI08,12,13,14; SI07,08,11; PC03; TH01,10; LU06; GB21; HT01,04.

Wrist, carpal pain, sprain, rheumatism, arthritis P: (Choose according to the affected channel and side): Ah Shi (local and shoulder girdle); LI04,05,06; SI04,05; TH04,05; HT05,07; PC07; LU07; S: SI06,11; TH06; LU08; A 09,22; T: SI03,05,08,10-14; LU06,09; LI03; HT06; PC04; TH02,03,13,14; BL12-17; BL41-46.

Metacarpal pain, sprain, rheumatism P: LI03,04; LU01,07; PC01,07,08; HT01,07; A 22; SI04; TH04; Ah Shi; S: LI05,06,11,20; LU05,08; SI03,07; TH02,03,05,23.

Finger (digital, upper limb) pain, sprain, rheumatism, arthritis P: Ah Shi; A 22; PC07; LU07; LI03,04; SI03,04,07; S: LI05; HT07; TH03,04,05; local periosteal acupuncture (Thumb: esp. LU07 and periosteal local acupuncture; Index: especially LI03,04,05; PC07; Middle: especially PC07,08; Fourth finger: esp. TH03; HT07; Little finger: especially SI07; TH03; HT07; T: LI06; HT03; TH06,13,14; A 09,17; PC04,06,08; GV14; SI06,08,10-14; BL12-17,41-6.

Disorders of the thoracic area, heart, lungs, trachea

Pain, trauma, rheumatism, stiffness, spasm, arthritis, slipped disc in thoracic spine and thoracic back muscle area P: Spinal Ah Shi; X 35; GV points, esp. 09,12,13,14; GB30; S: GV05,06,08,11; BL23,46,49,50; GB21,26; SI11,14; T: GV01,02,03,07,10,15,16; KI01,02,03,04,08; CV04,06,12,22; ST13,37,39,41; BL40,56,60,64; LI05; GB20,25; LU02; LV13.

Palpitations, atrial fibrillation, functional cardiac disorders P: HT05,07,09; PC06,07; BL15; S: HT06,08; PC03,05; BL10,14; CV14; T: HT03; PC04; BL11,12; LU04; LI04; ST36; LV01,03; GB20; CV06,12,17; GV24.

Bronchitis P: LU05; BL11,12,13,43; CV17,22; S: LU01; LI03; ST13,14,15,40; SI15; BL42,44; KI22,23; PC06; CV18,19,23; GV10,12,14; NX04; T: LU09; ST36; BL08,14,17; CV14; X 01; Acute P: LU05; BL13; CV22; LI04; GV14; S: PC06; TH05; BL12; ST40; GB20; T: LU07,08,09; LI06; SI17; BL10; SP06; GB21; CV17; GV16; Chronic P: LU05; BL13; CV22; ST40; CV12,17; BL12; S: PC06; BL08,20; LU06,07; CV06; GV12; LI04; T: LU01; ST36; BL11,17; CV18; NX04.

Asthma, bronchospasm, functional emphysema P: CV17,22; NX04; X 01; BL13; PC06; ST40; S: LU01,02,05,07,09,10; ST36; LI04; CV06,12; BL11; GV14; T: LU03,06,08; ST09,10,12,13,16; KI04,27; CV04,16,18,23; GV10,12; SI15; GB19,23,35,44; SP06.

Chronic rhinitis, sniffles P: LI04,20; Z 03,14; GB20; GV23,25; S: LI11,19; GV14,20,24; Z 15,16; BL07,08; LU05; GB04.

Soft moist cough, excess phlegm P: ST40; CV12; S: LU07; BL20; LI18.

Cough P: BL13; LU05,07; CV17,22; ST40; S: LU02,06,08,09,10,11; LI04; ST36; KI03,27; CV21; T: LU01,04; LI18; ST16; SP18; BL11,12,43; KI24,25,26; PC02; CV12,16,20; GV11,14.

Tracheitis (see laryngitis) P: CV22; BL11,13; S: LI04; GV14; ST40; LU05,07.

Disorders of abdominal area, digestive, reproductive, urinary systems and low back; disorders of the digestive tract

Malabsorption, ill-thrift, weight loss P: ST36; BL20,21; CV06; bleed A 09; S: CV12; KI03; LV13; BL17.

Anorexia, total inappetance P: ST36, KI17; CV12; S: CV10; GV07; ST21,22; SP04; HT07; BL20.

Poor appetite, inappetance P: BL20; ST36; S: KI17; CV12; GV07; ST22; SP06; HT07; BL18,21; LI04.

Digestive upsets, indigestion P: ST36; CV12; S: BL21; SP06; ST25; CV10; T: ST45; BL20,22,47,49; LV13,14; GV05,11; SP04,05,16; PC06; T: GV06,13,14; BL66; LI04; ST21,23; SP15,21.

Vomiting P: ST36; PC06; CV12; S: ST25; SP03,04; BL20,21; KI20; GV18; CV11,13,14,18,22; T: BL45,46,49,50; KI20,21,25,26; TH19; GB23; CV06,08,15,16; SI04; LV03,13; LI04; Neurogenic, nervous vomiting P: ST36; PC06; CV12; BL17.

Nausea P: PC06; CV12; ST36; S: HT03; BL21; CV02,03,13,14; Continuous: add KI01; Neurotic: add BL17; ST21.

Gastritis P: PC06; ST21,36; CV12,13; BL21; S: BL18,20; ST20,25; CV06; T: BL17,19,22; SP04,05,06; ST19,23,37.

Colic, gastric: *see* vomiting.

Enteritis P: BL22,25,29,53; GV05; S: ST25,36,37,39; BL21,27; CV06,08,10; GV03; SP05; Chronic: add Moxa CV08.

Gastroenteritis P: PC06; ST25,36; S: BL21; SP04; CV12; moxa CV08; needle points 0.5' near CV08; A 09 (4 points 1 inch near umbilicus).

Ulcerative colitis, colic, spasm P: ST25,36; SP15; CV06; BL25,27; S: CV12; BL20,21; LI04; HT07. T: LI10; ST17,28,37,40,44; HT03; BL22,24,31; PC06; GB28,34; LV03; CV03,04,08,13.

Diarrhoea P: ST25,36,37; CV04,06,12; SP04,06,09; BL20,25; LV13; S: ST34; moxa CV08; SP03,14,15; BL21; KI07; GV05,06; T: LI03,04: KI08,13,14,20,21; GV01,03; LV14; Chronic: add moxa CV08.

Constipation P: TH06; KI06; SP15 (or) ST25,26; CV06; BL25; SP03; KI16; S: CV12; BL27,28,33,36,38,50,51,57; SP03,16; GV01; GB34; T: ST40,44; CV03; LV01,02; LI02,11; GB28.

Colic (intestinal) P: ST25,36; CV06; moxa CV08; S: LI04; BL25; CV12;

LV03; T: ST37; LV02,05; SP14.

Paralytic ileus P: ST25,36; SP15; BL25,27.

Anal/perineal pruritus, pain P: GV01,20; BL57; SP10; S: BL25,32; TH06.

Tenesmus, anal ptosis, protrusion P: GV01,20; BL57; CV08 (moxa); S: GV02,06; CV06; ST25,36.

Disorders of the reproductive system

Pseudopregnancy (to terminate); to induce birth near term, misalliance (to abort) P: SP06; ST36; BL32; CV05,06; LI04; KI08; 'labour points' (2 inches lateral and 2 inches below umbilicus, bilateral; S: ST25; CV02; SP09.

Relaxation of pelvic ligaments in dystocia P: GV02,03,04; BL32,53; S: BL23,24,26,31,33,34,54.

To facilitate reposition of prolapsed uterus P: GV02,03,04; BL23,26,31,53; S: BL24,32,33,34,54.

Placental retention P: CV03; BL60,67.

Uterine inertia, failure to regress *post-partum* P: CV02,04; GV20; SP06; Y 16 to Y 18; S: ST29,36; CV03,06.

Lochiorrhoea P: CV07; Y 15.

Vaginal discharge, leucorrhea P: CV03,04,06; SP06; ST25; LV03; GB26; S: CV02,05; BL27,31-35; KI10,12; ST29; LV11; T: CV07; BL23,30; GV04; SP10; ST36; LV04.

Metritis P: BL30; SP12; GB26,27; S: BL27,28,31,32; GV04; CV07; GB28,29; T: BL25,33,35; SP06,10; ST29,36; LI04; CV02,03,04; Y 18.

Anoestrus, cystic ovaries, infertility P: Main point is 4 inches from mid-line in L5-L6 space (bilateral); use also Ah Shi points in lumbosacral area (i.e. in area BL23 to BL34); S: points from GV02,03,04; BL23,24,26,31-34,44,53.

Disorders of urinary system

Urinary tract disorders P: CV03,06; ST25; BL31-34; Ah Shi; S: CV04,05; SP06; LV08; BL23; GV04; X 35 (Sacral 1-4).

Bladder disorders P: CV03,06; SP06; BL23,28; S: BL32; CV04; SP09.

Cystitis P: BL28,38,58; CV03,04; KI02,03; ST28; S: BL23,25,26,31-33,54; GB26,29; SP06,09; CV02; T: ST27.

Bladder pain, spasm (in obstruction, calculi, colic) P: BL23,28; SP06; S: SP09; BL24,25,27,31,33; CV03,04,06; ST30,36

Dysuria, pain or difficulty on urination P: SP06,09; CV03,04; BL32; S: HT08; BL23,27,28,31,33,34,52; SP11; CV02,05,06,09; LV05,08; KI01,04,05,11; ST28,36; GV20.

Haematuria P: BL23,27; CV04,06; S: SP06; LV03; BL28; KI07.

Spastic bladder P: SP06; CV04; S: BL23; KI10; CV06; LV03.

Polyuria, diabetes insipidus P: BL23; CV04; S: GV04; BL21,22,24; LV13; CV03,06; SP06; KI07.

Urinary incontinence P: CV03,04; GV04; SP06; BL22,23; X 35 (L2-S5); S: CV02,06; GV20; BL25,27,28,67; LV01,02,03; KI02.

Bladder paralysis P: CV02,03,04; S: GV03; LV02; KI11; BL23,28,40.

Urine retention, postoperative urethral stricture, sphincter spasm; to evacuate bladder in cerebrovascular accident, stroke etc P: SP06; CV04; S: SP09; CV03; BL28; T: BL23,32,43; CV02; ST28.

Anuria, retention with coma, unconscious P: KI01; S: GV26.

Disorders of the lumbosacral area

Lumbar, loin, renal area, sacral area pain, rheumatism, stiffness, lowback syndrome, arthritis, spondylitis P: Ah Shi; X 35; BL23,25,27,31,40,52,60; GB30,38; GV02,03,04; S: BL22,24,26,32, 37,57; SI03; LV09; GV01; GB26,29,34; T: BL33,34,36,39,54,63,64,65; KI03,07; SP08; ST31; GB27.

Lower limb paralysis, posterior paralysis, paraplegia P: X 35; GB30,31,39; ST36; local points for region; GB34 to SP09; S: ST31,32,38,39,41,42; BL11,37,40,54,57,60; KI03; GB33; T: ST33,37,40; SP03,04,06; BL23,25,32,38,39,55,61,62; GB37,40,43; LV03,11; KI07,08; GV02,03; L 24.

Hip, thigh pain/rheumatism, arthritis etc P: Ah Shi; GB30,31,34; BL23,24; LV08,11; S: GB28,29,32,39; BL30,60; KI03.

Knee (stifle) pain, rheumatism, arthritis, etc P: Ah Shi; GB34 to SP09; GB33 to LV08; L 16 to L 16; GB30,38,39; ST33,35; BL40; S: ST34,36; LV07; BL57,60.

Ankle pain, strain, spavin, arthritis, rheumatism, etc. P: Ah Shi; BL60 to KI03; GB39,40; ST41; S: BL59,62,63; SP05,06; GB37.

Metatarsal pain, rheumatism, sprain, inflammation P: Ah Shi; BL60; ST42,43; L 05; S: BL57; ST41,44; KI03; LV03; T: GB34,39,41; SP04,05; KI06; LV02.

Toe pain, arthritis, rheumatism, etc. P: AhShi; L 08; SP04; LV03; S: ST41,43; GB34,40; BL60; KI03.

Acupuncture Analgesia

Abdominal surgery in adults: LU01 with TH08 to PC04.5 (i.e. between PC04 and PC05).

Abdominal surgery in children: BL23 (bilat) with ST36 (bilat) (or) SP06 to BL59 (bilateral).

Thoracic, head and upper limb surgery in children: Needle penetrating through the limb at level of PC06 and TH08 (both bilateral).

Inguinal and lower limb surgery in children: SP06 to BL59 (bilateral) +\- BL23 (bilateral).

APPENDIX 2
An introduction to Guang An Men Hospital

The Tao, considered as unchanging, has no name.

Tao Ti Ching

In China entire hospitals are dedicated to traditional Chinese medicine. Below is a report from such a hospital.

Guang An Men Hospital (including the Second Institute of Clinical Medicine and the Institute of Ophthalmology) was founded in 1955 as an affiliated hospital of China Academy of TCM. It is a general hospital of TCM conducting clinical practice, scientific research and teaching, together with specialities in many departments. It is a clinical pharmacological research base of Chinese herbs and also a part of the Traditional Medicine Co-operative centre organised by WHO. The State Administration Bureau of TCM awarded titles of 'The class A among First Grade of TCM Hospitals' and 'National Key Model Hospital of TCM' to Guang An Men Hospital in 1994. Entrusted by the Ministry of Public Health, this hospital runs TCM training courses for doctors of Western Medicine (WM).

Guang An Men Hospital boasts a large number of noted specialists in TCM and Integration of TCM and WM. They have contributed a lot to the development of TCM in China. At present, there are 816 medical and technical staff including 48 professors and 104 vice-professors. In addition, four TCM specialists have been awarded diplomas of 'Albert Einstein World Award of Science' by the World Cultural Council for their remarkable achievements in scientific research, four awarded national outstanding experts and special government prizes. In recent years 47 experts have become supervisors to postgraduates and 7 to candidates for doctorates. There are 13 wards with 505 beds in the Inpatient Department. The daily out patient visits number over 2,000. This hospital has 24 clinical departments including Internal Medicine, Surgery, Gynaecology, Paediatrics, Oncology, Ophthalmology, Orthopaedics, Acupuncture, Massage, Urology, Ch'i-gong, Proctology, Dermatology, Gerontology, Stomatology, ENT, Emergency and an Isolated dept. for patients of Hepatitis, 11 Medico-technical Depts. including pharmacy, Radiology, Clinical Lab, Ultrasonic Diagnosis Dept. Pathology, Endoscopic Dept. and Function Test Dept., one basic research room, one clinical pharmacological research room and 10 clinical research rooms including internal medicine, surgery, ophthalmology, orthopaedics, oncology, dermatology, urology, proctology, geriatrics and nursing dept.

This hospital now possesses all the modern equipment necessary for medical diagnosis, treatments and research, including CT, 200-1000mA X-Ray, Ultrasonic Technicolour Doppler, Flow Imaging System, Cranial Ultrasound, Abdominal Ultrasound, Bronchoscope, Gastroscope, Duodenoscope, Colonoscope, Holter, CCU, Automatic Biochemical Analyser, Hemodialysis and ESWL.

The characteristics of TCM are always emphasised in this hospital. Therefore, patients are mainly treated with traditional therapies, but are also supplemented with modern diagnostic methods. Rich experiences in developing effective therapies including acupuncture and massage have been accumulated in the treatments of cancer, cerebrocardiovascular diseases, diabetes mellitus, Bi syndrome (including rheumatic or rheumatoid arthritis), renal diseases, senile diseases, digestive diseases, retinal pigmentary degeneration, optic nerve atrophy, urinary stone, prostatic diseases, andropathy, psoriasis, eczema, soft tissue injury and common gynaecological and paediatric diseases. Since 1978, 55 scientific research achievements have been obtained. Among them, 3 belonged to national awards for scientific and technological progress, 16 were awarded by the Ministry of Public Health and 29 by the Academy of TCM. The well-known 'Xiao Zhi Ling' has won the gold medal of 14th Zagreb International Inventors Exhibition in Yugoslavia and the First Grade Knight Medal of the 35th Eureka World Inventors Exhibition in Brussels. This hospital has also invented a series of herbal patent medicine and health products of remarkable curative effects, such as 'Chinese Miraculous Recipe', pertaining to improve sexual potency, 'Hua Tai Nourishing Wine', 'No.1 Diabetic Conqueror Tablet', 'Diabetic Capsule to treat Vascular

Complication', 'Urinary Stone Expellent', 'Anti-prostatitis Pill', 'Psoriatic Conqueror Pill', 'Medicinal granules to invigorate the spleen and kidney' to treat cancers, 'Cold decoction to strengthen patient's resistance and to prevent cancerous growth', 'Anti-cancer and dephlogisticate capsule', 'Anti-asthmatic plaster', 'No.1 powder for external use to treat cervical erosion', 'No.1 Eyedrops for corneal virus infection' and 'Medicinal granules to treat arrhythmia'. The first two were elected as National New Products respectively by the National Science and Technology committee in 1991 and 1992.

Guang An Men Hospital has become an important window of international medical exchange. Each year foreigners from many countries come to the hospital for medical treatments, visits, study and academic exchange. Entrusted by the government, this hospital also provides medical service for foreigners at home and abroad. The international Clinical Acupuncture and TCM Training Centre has so far trained more than 1000 acupuncturists from many countries. At present, the basic course, advanced course and various training courses are organised to receive foreign learners of acupuncture, massage, internal medicine, herbs and Ch'i-gong (a system of deep breathing exercise).

Since the carrying out of the opening policy, as an experimental unit of the Ministry of Public Health, Guang An Men Hospital has been making some valuable exploration and much progress has been reached in various aspects, especially in medical treatments, research and education. All these achievements enable this hospital to enter into a new stage in its development. Emphasising 'the strategy of intellectuals, achievements, quality, characteristics and efficacy', as well as to cherish the hope of fully bringing out the potentialities, the staff of Guang An Men Hospital are working heart and soul to make their contribution advantageous to improve the health of people and to promote the development of TCM.

The characteristics of the main departments of Guang An Men Hospital

There are some famous TCM ophthalmologist in this clinic. They treat ophthalmology diseases by employing China herbs as the main therapeutic measures supplemented with Western medicine and have achieved good results. The project of treating cataract with needle snaring under the direction of Prof. Tang Youzhi won the Grade B Prize of National Scientific Progress. The rich experiences of treating diseases such as children's optic nerve atrophy, virus keratitis, pigmentary degeneration of retina have been accumulated.

Oncology Department

Oncology clinic is a centre of national TCM oncology speciality. The doctors in this clinic have done a lot of research in inhibiting oncology progress, reducing the side-effects of radio and chemical therapies, preventing recurring, improving the sufferers' QL and prolonging their life by employing integrated traditional and Western medicine. The 'Fu Zhen Chong-ji', 'Fei Liu Ping Gao', 'Fu Zhen Fang Ai Kou-fu-yie' and 'Jiao Wei Xi Huang Pill' etc. invented by them have good effects on preventing and treating the tumours of stomach, lung, liver, mammary gland, and rectum, and reducing the side-effects of radio and chemical therapies after surgery.

Anoprotology Department

Rich clinical experiences in treating haemorrhoid, rectum prolapse and ulcerative colitis, etc., have been achieved. The project of Xiao Zhi Ling injection in treating internal haemorrhoids under the direction of Prof. Shi Zhaoqi was awarded the grade B prize of National [LLK1] Science Progress in 1985 and twice awarded gold prizes at international fairs.

Urology Department

The doctors in this clinic, by employing integrated traditional and Western medicine, are good at treating prostate disease, and male sex disease etc. The project of relieving urolithiasis decoction conducted by Prof. Liu Youfang won the Grade C National Scientific Progress Prize.

Dermatology Department

The project of 'Ke Yin Fang in treating psoriasis under the direction of Prof. Zhu lenkang was awarded Grade A Scientific and Technological Achievement Prize of the Ministry of Public Health. The doctors in this clinic excel at treating lupus erythematosus, eczema, lichen planus, acne and baldness, etc.

Orthopaedics Department

The doctors in this department are good at treating cervical vertebral disease, lumbar intervertebral disc protrusion, osteoarthropathy and soft tissue injuries, etc.

Internal medicine clinics

The internal medicine clinics are divided into four divisions.

Internal medicine 1 is a specialised clinic for digestive diseases and rheumatic diseases. The doctors are good at treating rheumatic arthritis, rheumatoid arthritis, acute and chronic gastritis, peptic ulcer and oesophagis, etc.

Internal medicine 2 is a specialised clinic for diabetes and endocrine system diseases. The 'Jiang Tang Jiao tablet' and 'Jiang Tang Tong Mai tablet' invented by the doctors have good effect on diabetes and the vascular complications of diabetes. The study of the drugs mentioned above was awarded the grade B of the State Administration of TCM.

Internal medicine 3 is a specialised clinic for cardiovascular and respiratory diseases. The effects of 'Xiao Chuang Gao', treating asthma, 'Wen Xing Chongji' treating arrhythmia and tachycardia, 'Xing Kang Koufuyie', treating myocarditis are very good.

Internal medicine 4 is a specialised clinic for nephritis.

Geriatrics clinic is a specialised department for gerontological diseases such as amnesia, dementia, osteoporosis, fatty liver and hyperlipemia.

Acupuncture Department

Acupuncture is a traditional treatment therapy and has very good effects on over 100 diseases such as stroke, sequelae, pains, facial paralysis, diseases of the nervous system, myopia, hyperopia and strabismus, etc.

Gynaecology Department

The doctors in this clinic, by employing traditional Chinese medicine, are good at treating endometriosis, chronic pelvic inflammation and sterility etc. 'Gong Jing suppository 1' was awarded the grade C prize of Scientific Progress of SATCM.

Paediatrics Department

The 'Qiang Zhuang Ling' invented by the doctors was awarded the grade C prize of SATCM Scientific Progress and has good effect on child immune defect.

Emergency room

The Emergency room was founded in 1982. The doctors in this department have summarised a set of therapies integrated traditional Chinese and Western medicine treating the critically ill and improved the successful rate of saving the patient's life.

Pharmacology Department

The Pharmacology Department has divisions of Chinese herb preparation, Western medicine preparation, medicine examination, microbe examination, aseptic room and drug withdrawal workshop. The drug-produced clinical treatment and research amounts to 300 approximately.

Address: *Guang An Men Hospital, affiliated to China Academy of Traditional Chinese Medicine, Beijing, China 100053*
Tel: 86-010-63014195
Fax: 86-010-63014195

APPENDIX 3
An acupuncture survey

Simplicity without a name
Is free from all external aim.
With no desire, at rest and still,
All things go right as of their will.

Tao Ti Ching

The results of a survey conducted in the US recently came up with the following information. It is reproduced here merely for information and the reader should draw their own conclusions.

- 91.5% reported 'disappearance' or 'improvement' of symptoms after acupuncture treatment;
- 84% said they see their GPs less since receiving acupuncture;
- 79% said they use fewer prescription drugs;
- 70% of those to whom surgery had been recommended said they had avoided it;
- 63% of patients reported that they used acupuncture care to keep them healthy, most also reported that they used it to care for a wide range of complaints, ranging from depression to diabetes, from colds, sinus infections and allergies to neck and back pain, from HIV and hepatitis to insomnia, PMS, and infertility;
- 13.8% reported one or more complaints had disappeared;
- 77.7% said that some symptoms or complaints had improved;
- 7.8% named symptoms or conditions that had not changed;
- 0.7% said that a symptom or complaint had got worse;
- 57.0% said their improvement 'definitely' was due to acupuncture;
- 19.9% said it was 'probably' acupuncture;
- 17.5% said 'it was a combination of factors;
- there were more women than men (about two-thirds were women);

- most were middle-aged (ages 30–50 are the heaviest users);
- 89% were whites of European origin;
- most lived in urban or suburban settings;
- most had incomes in the US mid-range, neither poor nor wealthy, but with enough disposable income to pay for acupuncture care out-of-pocket;
- 22% had any insurance coverage for their acupuncture care;
- 22% had college degrees compared to 14.5% nationally;
- 51% had graduate education and/or graduate degrees, compared to 7.4% nationally;
- very likely to have professional and technical (38%) or entrepreneurial (14%) occupations. These two categories accounted for more than half of the respondents. Business people and blue-collar workers were under-represented;
- somewhat less likely than national averages to be married, and somewhat more likely to be single, living in unmarried partnerships, divorced, separated, or widowed;
- 80% of the respondents could report acupuncture costs accurately for the previous three months of acupuncture care. In three months, most patients saw their acupuncture practitioner six times or less. The average cost for all respondents for three months of visits was $238.52 (combining all sites, including the lower costs of school clinics with the usually higher costs of private clinics);
- 84% said they were seeing their GP less;
- 58.5% said they were seeing a psychotherapist less;
- 77.5% said they were seeing a physical therapist less;
- 78.9% said they had reduced the use of prescription drugs;
- 77% reported they were asking for fewer reimbursements from their insurance company;
- 70.1% of the respondents who said they had been recommended surgery before acupuncture treatment said they had avoided surgery subsequent to receiving acupuncture care. These were not minor surgeries. Respondents reported avoiding back surgery and several types of abdominal surgery, as well as milder oral or skin surgeries;
- 72% reported they had never experienced harm from the needles;
- 24.6% said they had experienced a small bruise or a drop of blood at the needle site;
- 3.6% said they had experienced something more serious, such as a pimple or rash;
- The great majority of respondents reported that their practitioners use only sterile, disposable needles. Only 8.3% reported they were treated with reusable needles.

APPENDIX 4
Common ailments and their treatments

Without going outside the door, one understands (all that takes place) under the sky; without looking out from the window, one sees the Tao of Heaven. The farther that one goes out the less one knows.

Tao Ti Ching

Abscesses

Source: Heat and fire poison in the blood.
Treatment: Internally a tea made from violet, wild chrysanthemum or dandelion and Chinese golden thread; externally, peony flowers or rhubarb crushed and mixed with oil as a ointment

Acid stomach

Source: Deficient spleen, imbalance of liver and spleen.
Treatment: Tonify spleen, dry dampness and soothe the liver, reduce stagnation.
Use: Ginseng, liquorice, tangerine peel.
Avoid: Cold food, acidic food.

Acne

Source: Excess heat in the blood and stomach.
Use: Herbal teas of chrysanthemum, dandelion and honeysuckle. Externally cucumber and watermelon juice.

Alcoholism

Source: Excess heat.
Treatment: Clear heat from blood and liver.
Use: Watermelon or Kudzu vine to detoxify blood.

Amnesia

Source: Kidney weakness.
Use: Wolfberry seed, mulberry fruit, eucommia bark, bodder seed.

Anaemia

Source: Spleen not transforming ch'i properly.
Treatment: Gui Pi Wan (Return Spleen Tablets).

Angina

Source: Stagnating ch'i in the blood and heart.
Treatment: Safflower, cinnamon twigs, red sage root, peony root, macrosten onion bulb.
Note: This condition is serious and should not be treated at home. Consult a qualified practitioner.

Anorexia

Source: Weakness of stomach and spleen.
Use: Wheat sprouts, rice sprouts, loganberries, radish seeds.

Anxiety

Source: Weakness of the spleen, depression of liver ch'i.
Treatment: Strengthen spleen and enliven liver ch'i.
Use: Ginseng, Chinese angelica. White peony root with thorowax root for relaxation.

Arthritis

Source: Wind damp. Painful joints are caused by wind cold.
Use: Cinnamon twigs to release the ch'i, aconite root, angelica root and wild ginger to relieve the cold and damp.
Note: If there are not painful joints it is regarded as wind heat

because the joints are usually swollen and hot. Use large leafed gentian and corktree bark.

Asthma

Source: Phlegm produced by a weakness of the spleen and kidneys.
Treatment: Bitter almond seed and ephedra to open up the lung passages.
Note: there are many causes of asthma. Seek qualified diagnosis.

Back pain

Source: Too many to list, including physical injury.
Treatment: Acupuncture, massage, Qi Gong.
Use: Teasel root, ginseng and acanthopanax root to relieve pain.

Bed-wetting

Source: Weak kidney ch'i
Use: Dried chicken gizzard, walnut and black ginger seeds to tonify the kidneys.

Blood-pressure

Source: High blood-pressure is regarded as internal wind.
Treatment: Liver yin and blood wind calmed with peony root, chrysanthemum flowers and astralagus.
Source: Low blood-pressure is regarded as deficient ch'i in the blood and heart.
Use: Ginseng and Chinese angelica.

Bronchitis

Source: (Acute) External wind, cold or heat; (chronic) internal deficient spleen or lungs or internal mucus.
Use: (Acute) Fritillary bulb, plantain seed and balloon flower root; (Chronic) honeysuckle flowers, mulberry leaf and gardenia fruit.

Cancer

Source: Deficient ch'i, blood yin or yang.
Treatment: Consult qualified practitioner.

Candida

Source: Dampness in the blood.
Use: Poria, magnolia bark and pinellia tube.
Avoid: Dairy products and sugar.

Cataracts

Source: Weak liver and kidneys due to deficient blood.
Use: Wolfberry, chrysanthemum flowers, rumania and dendronbrum.

Catarrh

Sources: Many.
Use: Blackberry leaves, peppermint and magnolia flowers. Use ginger and orange peel in food.

Chickenpox

Source: Wind and heat invasion.
Use: Safflowers, cimicifuga and honeysuckle.

Chilblains

Source: Yang ch'i deficient.
Use: Cinnamon twigs, red sage, angelica, dried ginger and aconite root.

Chills

Source: External cold (can be a symptom of the onset of more serious condition).
Use: Ginger.

Cystitis

Source: Damp heat
Use: Plantain.

Deafness

Source: Many, including physical injury.
Treatment: Consult practitioner to find out the cause.

Depression

Source: Stagnation of liver ch'i.
Use: Angelica, peony root, liquorice and thorowax root.

Diabetes

Source: Sweet urine disease, yin deficient heat lung disorder.
Treatment: To help nourish the spleen, kidneys and stomach use Chinese yam, lotus seed and mulberry. Insulin-dependent diabetics must see a practitioner before administering any self-remedy.

Diarrhoea

Source: Many and varied.
Use: Acute – skullcap root, golden thread, kapok flowers and dandelion. Chronic – psoralea fruit, codonopsis root and astragulus.

Dizziness

Source: Chronic – kidney deficient or liver heat in cases of high blood-pressure; Acute – wind invasion in cases after illness such as influenza.
Use: Fresh ginger, cinnamon twigs and peppermint. For nourishing blood use mulberry.

Dysentery

Source: Damp heat external.
Use: Peony root, skullcap root, golden thread and anemone.

Eczema

Source: Open weeping – damp heat. Dry red – excess heat in blood. Allergic – wind.
Use: For allergic eczema use ledebouriella root and schizonepeta or peony root, Chinese gentian and rumania. See practitioner for the other types.

Epilepsy

Source: Excess heart mucus, internal damp, stagnant ch'i or blood.
Treatment: Consult a practitioner.

Use: Sweet flag root and the juice from young bamboo can sometimes cut down the number of attacks.

Exhaustion

Source: Deficient ch'i or blood.
Use: Ginseng and astragulus.

Eyesight

Source: Exhausted blood.
Use: Wolfberry, mulberry, chrysanthemum flowers and cassia seed.

Flatulence

Source: Stagnant stomach ch'i or damp heat.
Use: Orange peel, perilla stem and magnolia bark.

Frozen shoulder

Source: Weak yang ch'i, external cold and damp.
Treatment: Acupuncture.
Use: Cinnamon twigs and turmeric.

Hair loss

Source: Deficient liver and kidneys.
Use: Wolfberry, mulberry and fleece flower root.

Halitosis

Source: Stomach damp heat.
Use: Golden thread, peppermint tea, giant hyssop and radish seeds.

Hepatitis A (acute)

Source: Excess liver and gall bladder damp heat.
Treatment: Consult practitioner.
Use: Gardenia fruit and oriental wormwood.

Hepatitis B (viral)

Source: Deficient ch'i, weakened liver.
Treatment: Consult a practitioner.
Use: Peony root, mulberry, ginseng, liquorice and astragulus.

Hiccups

Source: Heat, cold or food stagnation.
Use: Berilla stems, rhubarb and ginger.

Impotence

Source: Weakness of kidneys and liver, liver ch'i stagnation.
Use: Sea-horse and cibot root.

Incontinence

Source: Kidney yang deficiency with internal cold.
Use: Golden lock tea.

Indigestion

Source: Weakness of spleen and stomach.
Use: Rice and wheat sprouts and chicken gizzards (*see* Bed-wetting).

Infertility

Source: Damp heat, yin–yang imbalance.
Treatment: Consult practitioner.

Influenza

Source: Wind cold, damp, wind heat.
Treatment: Moxibustion.
Use: Honeysuckle, peppermint, chrysanthemum and cinnamon.

Insomnia

Source: Heat in the heart driving out Shen, weakness in the kidneys, overeating.
Treatment: Massage, acupressure and exercise.

Use: Poria, fleece flower stem and wild jujubes. Sleeping on a gypsum pillow.

Irritable bowel syndrome

Source: Weakness of kidneys and spleen, excess dampness in intestines, liver ch'i stagnation.
Use: Dandelion, rhubarb, magnolia and angelica.

Itching

Source: External or internal wind.
Use: Dittnay bark, puncture vine fruit.

Jaundice

Source: Dampness in gall bladder and liver.
Treatment: Consult a practitioner.
Use: Gardenia fruit, oriental wormwood and corktree bark.

Laryngitis

Source: Poisoned heat in lungs.
Use: Peppermint, honeysuckle flowers, mulberry, lily and liquorice.

Leukaemia

Treatment: Consult practitioner.

Ligaments (torn and sprained)

Source: Internal blood and ch'i stagnation.
Treatment: Acupuncture, massage and herbal plasters.
Use: Safflower, ginseng and millettia stem.

Lumbago

Source: Many, including physical injury. Excess internal cold.
Use: A tincture of achyranthes root and acanthopanax bark in alcohol.

Malaria

Source: Internal and external simultaneously.
Use: Bupleurum Tonic and Seven Wonder Tonic. It could well be necessary to add or subtract ingredients.

Mastitis

Source: Stagnant ch'i and blood.
Use: Peony bark, dandelion, Chinese gentian and madder root.

ME (Myalgic Encephalomyelitis)

Source: Weakness of ch'i, deficient blood, damp heat.
Treatment: Responds well to acupuncture.

Measles

Source: Excess heat in blood and stomach.
Use: Peppermint, safflowers and honeysuckle.

Memory loss

Source: Deficient kidney essence.
Use: Dodder seeds, mulberry and black ginger seeds.

Menopause

Source: Weakness of the kidneys, deficient blood and kidney–liver imbalance between kidney and liver.
Use: Angelica, peony root and thorowax root.

Menstrual problems

Source: Excessive blood loss – heat in blood. Scanty blood flow – cold in blood. Late periods – cold in blood. Painful periods – Cold in blood.
Treatment: Acupuncture, moxibustion.

Migraine

Source: Excess liver ch'i stagnation, weakness in stomach.
Stomach–liver imbalance.

Treatment: Acupuncture, consult practitioner.
Use: Chrysanthemum, cassiae torae.

Morning sickness

Source: Excess cold. Weakness of the stomach.
Use: Fresh ginger, ginger tea.
Avoid: Cold foods.

Mosquito bites

Source: Poisoned blood.
Use: Palm oil applied externally.

Mumps

Source: Wind, damp heat.
Use: Dandelion, honeysuckle, skullcap and rhubarb.

Nausea

Source: Ascending stomach ch'i.
Treatment: Acupressure.

Nephritis

Source: Heat invading lung, weakness of spleen, deficient kidneys.
Treatment: Consult practitioner.

Nettle-rash

Source: Heat and wind when rash is red and hot, cold and wind when rash is cold and white.
Use: Schizomeotea, ledebouriella.

Neuritis

Source: Wind, damp and heat invading meridians.
Treatment: Consult practitioner.

Nose and throat conditions

Source: Weakness of lung, cold and wind.
Use: Plaintain seed, peppermint, mulberry, honeysuckle and skullcap.

Nosebleed

Source: Heat in the blood.
Use: Peony roots, thistles, romania.

Obesity

Source: Excess mucus and dampness, weakened spleen.
Treatment: Acupuncture, exercise, Ch'i Kung. Consult practitioner.

Oedema

Source: Excess water, kidney deficiency.
Use: Ginseng, water plaintain, poria, cinnamon twigs, Ephedra.

Osteoarthritis

Source: Weakness in the kidneys, blood stagnation.
Use: Ledebouriellus root, cinnamon twigs, timospra stem, angelica.
Avoid: Cold.

Osteoporosis

Source: Kidney deficiency.
Use: Cibote rhizome, drynaria tuber, eucomia bark.

Palpitations

Source: Heart blood deficiency.
Treatment: Acupuncture.
Use: Asparagus root, wild jujube seed.

Parkinson's disease

Source: Deficient blood, deficient kidney yin.
Treatment: Acupuncture.
Use: Gastrodia tube, peony root, peony buds, wolfberry root.

Peptic ulcer

Source: Stagnating stomach ch'i, weakness of the spleen, excess heat.
Use: Ginseng, dandelion, corvdalis tube.
Avoid: Cold food, alcohol, coffee, tea.

Phlebitis

Source: Excess heat in the blood.
Use: Golden thread, peony bark, safflower, rhubarb root.

Pimples and spots: *see* Acne

Pink eye

Source: Wind heat in liver meridians.
Use: Boil bamboo leaves, violets and chrysanthemum flowers, and use the cooled water to bathe eyes.

Pneumonia

Source: Mucus and heat in the lung.
Treatment: Consult practitioner.
Use: Peach kernel, skullcap, fritillary bulb.

Poliomyelitis

Source: Weak ch'i and blood.
Treatment: Acupuncture. Consult practitioner.

Pre-menstrual syndrome

Source: Imbalance of spleen, kidneys and liver.
Use: Angelica, skullcap, poria, peony.

Prolapse

Source: Deficient ch'i.
Use: Central ch'i pills.

Prostate problems

Source: Excess dampness, stagnant ch'i.
Use: Cinnamon bark, corktree bark, water plaintain.

Quinsy

Source: Fire and heat poison in the blood.
Use: Golden thread, dandelion, skullcap, forsythia fruit.

Rheumatism

Source: Ch'i stagnation, excess wind, damp and heat.
Use: Achyranthes root and corktree bark.

Rheumatoid arthritis

Source: Excess internal coldness.
Treatment: Acupuncture.
Use: Powdered rhubarb and sesame oil.

Rubella

Source: External wind, heat.
Use: Mulberry, honeysuckle, chrysanthemum.

Sciatica

Source: Heat stagnation in the gall bladder.
Treatment: Acupuncture

Scrofula

Source: Liver and kidney yin deficiency.
Use: Gardenia fruit, fritillary bulb, eclipta.

Seasickness

Source: External movement.
Use: Fresh ginger.

Shingles

Source: Gall bladder heat and damp.
Use: Gentian and oriental wormwood.

Sinusitis

Source: Lung ch'i deficient.
Use: Honeysuckle, peppermint, fritillary bulb.

Spastic colon

Source: Excess cold, stagnant ch'i, weak blood.
Use: Fresh ginger, cinnamon twigs, peony, astragulus.

Stroke

Source: Wind stroke
Treatment: Consult practitioner, acupuncture.

Sweating

Source: Deficient ch'i, yin deficiency.
Use: For ch'i deficiency use ledebourella and astragulus. For yin deficiency use lilyturf root, corktree bark and peony.

Tennis elbow

Source: Cold and damp in the elbow.
Use: Mulberry twigs, cinnamon twigs, angelica root and ginger.

Thrush

Source: Excess damp, damp heat.
Use: Gentian and oriental wormwood.

Tonsillitis

Source: Fire poison, wind and heat.
Use: Honeysuckle tea.
Avoid: Spicy food.

Toothache

Source: Heat in the stomach, decayed or damaged teeth.
Treatment: Visit dentist, acupuncture.
Use: Gypsum to relieve the heat, ginseng.

Ulcerated colitis

Source: Poisoned blood, excess damp.
Use: Dandelion, astragulus.

Varicose veins

Source: Bad circulation, stagnant ch'i or blood.
Use: Internally, angelica, cinnamon twigs, astragulus; Externally, honey.

Vertigo

Source: Blood deficiency, deficient ch'i, liver wind.
Treatment: Consult practitioner.

Caution

Anyone with persistent or serious symptoms should consult their GP or a qualified practitioner of Chinese herbal medicine. Self-diagnosis and self-treatment are not to be recommended or advised except for the most minor of conditions.

APPENDIX 5
Chinese herbal
medicine

The great Tao (or way) is very level and easy; but people love the
by-ways.

Tao Ti Ching

Conditions treated and Chinese names for herbal formulas

Tonify yin	Bai He Gu Jin Tang
Tonify yin	Liu Wei Di Huang Wan
Tonify yin	Liu Wei Di Huang Wan Jiu
Tonify yin	Ch'i Ju Di Huang Wan
Tonify yin	Ch'i Wei Du Ch'i Wan
Tonify yin	Yi Guan Jian Jiu
Tonify yin	Zhi Bai Di Huang an
Tonify yin	Zuo Gui Yin Jiu
Tonify yin	Mai Men Dong Tang
Tonify yang	Du Zhong Bu Tian Su
Tonify yang	Jin Kui Di Huang Wan
Tonify yang	Jin Suo Gu Jing Wan
Tonify yang	Li Zhong Wan
Tonify yang	Qing Chun Bao
Tonify yang	Yao Tong Pian
Tonify yang	Zhuang Yao Jian Shen Pian
Tonify ch'i and blood	B Zhen Tang Jiu
Tonify ch'i and blood	Ren Shen Yang Rong Tang Jiu
Tonify ch'i and blood	Shi Quan Da Bu Tang Jiu
Tonify ch'i	Bu Zhong Yi Ch'i Tang
Tonify ch'i	Bu Zhong Yi Ch'i Tang Jiu
Tonify ch'i	Bu Zhong Yi Ch'i Wan
Tonify ch'i	Liu Jun Zi Pian

Tonify ch'i	Liu Jun Zi Tang
Tonify ch'i	Liu Jun Zi Tang Jiu
Tonify ch'i	Ch'i Wei Bai Zu San Jiu
Tonify ch'i	Shen Ling Bai Zhu Pian
Tonify ch'i	Shen Ling Bai Zhu San
Tonify ch'i	Shen Ch'i Da Bu Wan
Tonify ch'i	Si Jian Zi Tang
Tonify ch'i	Si Jun Zi Tang Jiu
Tonify ch'i	Zi Sheng Wan
Tonify both ch'i and blood	Ba Zhen Tang
Tonify both ch'i and blood	Ba Zhen Wan
Tonify both ch'i and blood	Gui Pi Tang
Tonify both ch'i and blood	Gui Pi Wan
Tonify both ch'i and blood	Huang Jiang Hua Fen
Tonify both ch'i and blood	Shi Quan Da Bu Wan
Tonify both ch'i and blood	Shi Quan Da Bu Wan
Tonify both ch'i and blood	Shuang Bao Su
Tonify both ch'i and blood	Yang Rong Wan
Tonify both ch'i and blood	Zhi Gan Cao Tang
Tonify both ch'i and blood	Ren Shen Yang Rong Tang
Tonify blood	Dang Gui Bu Xue Tang Jiu
Tonify blood	Dang Gui Pian Jiu
Tonify blood	Gui Pi Tang Jiu
Tonify blood	Si Wu Tang Jiu
Subdue wind	Gou Teng San
Subdue wind	Wu Yao Shun Ch'i San
Subdue wind	Xiao Feng San
Subdue wind	Xu Ming Tang
Subdue wind	Yi Gan San
Subdue internal wind	Fu Fang Du Zhong Pian
Subdue internal wind	Jian Ya Wan
Subdue internal wind	Jiang Ya Ping Pian
Subdue internal wind	Tian Ma Qui Feng Bu Pian
Resolve Tan	Ban Xia Bai Zhu Tian Ma Tang
Resolve Tan	Bu Fei Tang Jiu
Resolve Tan	Chuan Bei Pi Pa Lu
Resolve Tan	Ding Chuan Tang
Resolve Tan	Er Chen Tang
Resolve Tan	Er Chen Tang Jiu
Resolve Tan	Er Chen Wan
Resolve Tan	Jie Geng Wan
Resolve Tan	Ling Gan Wu Wei Jiang Xin Tang

Resolve Tan	Nei Xiao Luo Li Wan
Resolve Tan	Ning Sou Wan
Resolve Tan	Ping Chuan Wan
Resolve Tan	Qing Ch'i Hua Tan Wan
Resolve Tan	Suzi Jiang Ch'i Tang
Resolve Tan	Tong Xuan Li Fei Wan
Resolve Tan	Wen Dan Tang
Resolve Tan	Xiao Qing Long Tang
Resolve Tan	Xing Su San
Resolve Tan	Zhi Sou San
Resolve Tan	Ping Wei Pian
Regulate ch'i	Ban Xia Hou Po Tang Jui
Regulate ch'i	Gua Lou Xie Bai Jiu Tang Jiu
Regulate ch'i	Ju Pi Zhu Ru Tang Jiu
Regulate ch'i	Shu Gan Wan
Regulate ch'i	Su Zi Jiang Ch'i Tang Jiu
Regulate ch'i	Xiang Sha Liu Jun Wan
Regulate ch'i	Xiang Sha Yang Wei Pian
Regulate ch'i	Xiao Yao Wan
Regulate ch'i	Zhi Shi Gua Lou Gui Zhi Tang Jiu
Regulate blood	Ba Li San
Regulate blood	Da Huang Mu Dan Tang
Regulate blood	Dan Shen Yin Jiu
Regulate blood	Fu Fang Dan Shen Pian
Regulate blood	Fu Yuan Huo Xue Tang
Regulate blood	Guan Xin Su He Wan
Regulate blood	Gui Zhi Fu Ling Wan
Regulate blood	Gui Zhi Fu Ling Wan Jiu
Regulate blood	Huo Luo Xiao Ling Dan Jiu
Regulate blood	Sheng Hua Tang
Regulate blood	Sheng Hua Tang Jiu
Regulate blood	Shu Jing Huo Xue Tang
Regulate blood	Tao He Cheng Ch'i Tang
Regulate blood	Tao Hong Si Wu Tang Jiu
Regulate blood	Tong Jing Wan
Regulate blood	Wei Te Ling
Regulate blood	Wen Jing Tang
Regulate blood	Wen Jing Tang Jiu
Regulate blood	Xian Fang Huo Ming Yin
Regulate blood	Xiong Gui Jiao Ai Tang
Regulate blood	Yun Nan Bai Yao
Regulate blood	Yun Nan Te Chan Tian Ch'i Pian

Reduce food stagnation	Bao Jian Mei Jian Fei Cha
Reduce food stagnation	Jian Pi Wan
Reduce food stagnation	Shen Qu Cha
Protect Wei ch'i	Yu Ping Feng San Jiu
Nourish yin	Ba Xian Chang Shou Wan
Nourish yin	Da Bu Yin Wan
Nourish yin	Gu Ben Wan
Nourish yin	Jie Wan
Nourish yin	Jin Mu Li
Nourish yin	Liu Wei Di Huang Wan
Nourish yin	Ming Mu Di Huang Wan
Nourish yin	Ch'i Ju di Huang Wan
Nourish yin	Run Chang Wan
Nourish yin	Zhi Bai Ba Wei Wan
Nourish blood	Dang Gu Su
Nourish blood	Dang Cui Pian
Nourish blood	Dang Gui Shao Yao San
Nourish blood	Dang Gui Wan
Nourish blood	Fu Ke Zhong Zi Wan
Nourish blood	Shao Yao Gan Cao Tang
Nourish blood	Shou Wu Pian
Nourish blood	Si Wu Tang
Nourish blood	Wen Qing Yin
Nourish blood	Er Ming Zuo Chi Wan
Nourish blood	Dang Gui San
Harmonise / regulate ch'i	Xiao Chai Hu Tang
Harmonise / regulate ch'i	Gan Cao Xie Xin Tang
Harmonise / regulate ch'i	Ban Xia Hou Po Tang
Harmonise / regulate ch'i	Ban Xia Xie Xin Tang
Harmonise / regulate ch'i	Chai Hu Gui Jiang Tang
Harmonise / regulate ch'i	Chai Hu Gui Zhi Tang
Harmonise / regulate ch'i	Chai Hu Xian Xiong Tang
Harmonise / regulate ch'i	Da Chai Hu Tang
Harmonise / regulate ch'i	Hou Po Ch'i Wu Tang
Harmonise / regulate ch'i	Huang Lian Tang
Harmonise / regulate ch'i	Jia Wei Xio Yao San
Harmonise / regulate ch'i	Shen Mi Tang
Harmonise / regulate ch'i	Sheng Jiang Xie Xin Tang
Harmonise / regulate ch'i	Si Ni San
Harmonise / regulate ch'i	Wu Ji San
Harmonise / regulate ch'i	Xiang Sha Yang Wei Tang
Harmonise / regulate ch'i	Xiang Sha Liu Jun Zi Tang

Harmonise / regulate ch'i	Xiao Yao San
Harmonise and regulate	Chai Hu Shu Gan Tang Jiu
Harmonise and regulate	Xiao Yao San Jiu
Harmonise and regulate	Si Ni San Jiu
Flush downwards	Da Cheng Ch'i Tang
Flush downwards	Fang Feng Tong Sheng San
Flush downwards	Liang Ge San
Flush downwards	Ma Zi Ren Wan
Flush downwards	Run Chang Wan
Flush downwards	Tiao Wei Cheng Ch'i Tang
Flush downwards	Xiao Cheng Ch'i Tang
Firm and gather	Fu Tu Dan
Firm and gather	Gui Zhi Jia Long Gu Mu Li Tang
Firm and gather	Jin Suo Gu Jing Wan
Firm and gather	Sang Piao Xiao San
External use	Die Da Yao Jing Liniment
External use	Yun Nan Bai Yao Plasters
External use	Zheng Gu Shui Liniment
Expel wind–heat	Cha Ge Jie Ji Tang
Expel wind–heat	Sang Ju Yin
Expel wind–heat	Sheng Ma Ge Gen Tang
Expel wind–heat	Yi Ch'i Cong Ming Tang
Expel wind-heat	Yin Qiao San
Expel wind–cold	Cang Er San
Expel wind–cold	Chuan Xiong Cha Tiao San
Expel wind–cold	Da Qing Long tang
Expel wind–cold	Ge Gen Tang
Expel wind–cold	Gui Zhi Jia Shao Yao Tang
Expel wind–cold	Gui Zhi Tang
Expel wind–cold	Hua Gai san
Expel wind–cold	Jing Fang Bai Du San
Expel wind–cold	Jiu Wei Qiang Huo Tang
Expel wind–cold	Ma Huang Tang
Expel wind–cold	Ren Shen Bai Du San
Expel wind–cold	Shen Su Yin
Expel wind–cold	Shi Wei Xiang Ru Yin
Expel wind–cold	Xiang Su San
Expel wind–cold	Xin Yi San
Expel external wind	Bi Yan Pian
Expel external wind	Cang Er San Jiu
Expel external wind	Chuan Xiong Cha Tiao Wan
Expel external wind	Gan Mao Ling

Expel external wind	Gan Mao Qing Re Chong Ji
Expel external wind	Yin Qiao Wan
Expel damp	Ba Zheng San
Expel damp	Bao He Wan
Expel damp	Bi Xie Fen Qing Yin
Expel damp	Bi Xie Fen Qing Yin
Expel damp	Dao Shu Fu Ling Tang
Expel damp	Du Huo Ji Sheng Tang
Expel damp	Du Huo Ji Sheng Wan
Expel damp	Fang Ji Huang Ch'i Tang
Expel damp	Fen Xiao Tang
Expel damp	Huo Xiang Zheng Ch'i Pian
Expel damp	Kang Ning Wan
Expel damp	Liu He Tang
Expel damp	Ma Xing Yi Gan Tang
Expel damp	Ping Wei San
Expel damp	Te Xiao Yao Tong Ling
Expel damp	Wei Ling Tang
Expel damp	Wu Lin San
Expel damp	Wu Ling San
Expel damp	Wu Pi Yin
Expel damp	Yi Ren Tang
Expel damp	Yin Chen Wu Ling San
Expel damp	Yue Bi Jia Zhu Tang
Expel damp	Zhu Ling Tang
Expel damp	Huo Xiang Zheng Ch'i San
(External use)	Qing Liang You
Eliminate wind-damp	Du Huo Ji Sheng Tang Jiu
Eliminate wind-damp	Juan Bi Tang Jiu
Eliminate wind-damp	Qiang Huo Sheng Shi Tang Jiu
Eliminate dampness	Ping Wei San Jiu
Eliminate dampness	San Miao San Jiu
Clear heat and fire	Long Dan Xie Gan Tang Jiu
Clear heat	Bai Hu Jia Ren Shen Tang
Clear heat	Bai Hui Tang
Clear heat	Bai Tou Weng Tang
Clear heat	Cai Feng Zhen Zhu An Chuang Wan
Clear heat	Chai Hu Qing Gan Tang
Clear heat	Dao Chi Pian
Clear heat	Dao Chi San
Clear heat	Huang Lian Jie Du Tang

Clear heat	Huang Qin Tang
Clear heat	Li Dan Pian
Clear heat	Lian Qiao Bai Du Pian
Clear heat	Long Dan Xie Gan Wan
Clear heat	Long Dian Xie Gan Tang
Clear heat	Ma Xing Gan Shi Tang
Clear heat	Qin Jiao Rue Jia San
Clear heat	Qing Shiu YI Ch'i Tang
Clear heat	Qing Wei San
Clear heat	Qing Zao Jiu Fei Tang
Clear heat	San Huang Shi Gao Tang
Clear heat	Shao Yao Tang
Clear heat	Sun Huang Xie Xin Tang
Clear heat	Xie Bai San
Clear heat	Xing Jiu Ling
Clear heat	Yin Chen Hao Tang
Clear heat	Yu Nu Jian
Clear heat	Zhen Zhu San
Clear heat	Zhu Ye Shi Gao Tang
Calm Shen	An Shen Bu Xin Wan
Calm Shen	Bai Zi Yang Xin Wan
Calm Shen	Chai Hu Jia Long Gu Mu Li Tang
Calm Shen	Gan Mai Da Zao Tang
Calm Shen	Shui Mina Ning
Calm Shen	Suan Zao Ren Tang
Calm Shen	Suan Zao Ren Tang Jiu
Calm Shen	Suan Zao Ren Tang Pian
Calm Shen	Tian Wang Bu Xin Dan
Calm Shen	Tian Wang Bu Xin Dan Jiu
Calm Shen	Tian Wang Bu Xin Wan
Calm Shen	Yang Xin Tang

APPENDIX 6
Acupuncture points, with Chinese names

From above it is not bright;
From below it is not dark:
Unbroken thread beyond description.
It returns to nothingness.
Form of the formless,
Image of the imageless,
It is called indefinable and beyond imagination.

Tao Ti Ching

Bl 1 (Bl 1): III 1: jing ming
Bl 2 (Bl 2): III 2: an zhu
Bl 7 (Bl 7): III 7: tong tian
Bl 10: III 10: tian zhu
Bl 11: III 11: da zhu
Bl 12: III 12: feng men
Bl 13: III 13: fei shu
Bl 14: III 14: jue yin shu
Bl 15: III 15: xin shu
Bl 16: III 16: du shu
Bl 17: III 17: ge shu
Bl 18: III 18: gan shu
Bl 19: III 19: dan shu
Bl 20: III 20: pi shu
Bl 21: III 21: wei shu
Bl 22: III 22: san jiao shu
Bl 23: III 23: shen shu
Bl 24: III 24: ch'i hai shu
Bl 25: III 25: da chang shu

Bl 26: III 26: guan yuan shu
Bl 27: III 27: xiao chang shu
Bl 28: III 28: pang guang shu
Bl 29: III 29: zhong lu shu
Bl 30: III 30: bai huan shu
Bl 31: III 31: shang liao
Bl 32: III 32: ci liao
Bl 33: III 33: zhong liao
Bl 34: III 34: xia liao
Bl 35: III 35: hui yang
Bl 36: III 36: fu fen
Bl 37: III 37: po hu
Bl 38: III 38: gao huang shu
Bl 39: III 39: shen tang
Bl 40: III 40: yi xi
Bl 41: III 41: ge guan
Bl 42: III 42: hun men
Bl 43: III 43: yang gang
Bl 44: III 44: yi she

Bl 45: III 45: wei cang
Bl 46: III 46: huang men
Bl 47: III 47: zhi shi
Bl 48: III 48: bao huang
Bl 49: III 49: zhi bian
Bl 53: III 53: wei yang
Bl 54: III 54: wei zhong
Bl 57: III 57: cheng shan
Bl 58: III 58: fei yang
Bl 59: III 59: fu yang
Bl 60: III 60: kun lun
Bl 61: III 61: pu can
Bl 62: III 62: shen mai
Bl 63: III 63: jin men
Bl 64: III 64: jing gu
Bl 65: III 65: shu gu
Bl 66: III 66: zu tong gu
Bl 67: III 67: zhi yin
CV 1 (CV 1): XIII 1: hui yin
CV 2 (CV 2): XIII 2: qu gu
CV 3 (CV 3): XIII 3: zhong ji
CV 4 (CV 4): XIII 4: guan yuan
CV 5 (CV 5): XIII 5: shi men
CV 6 (CV 6): XIII 6: ch'i hai
CV 7 (CV 7): XIII 7: yin jiao
CV 8 (CV 8): XIII 8: ch'i zhong
CV 9 (CV 9): XIII 9: shui fen
CV 10: XIII 10: xia guan
CV 11: XIII 11: jian li
CV 12: XIII 12: zhong wan
CV 13: XIII 13: shang wan
CV 14: XIII 14: ju que
CV 15: XIII 15: jiu wei
CV 17: XIII 17: shan zhong
CV 21: XIII 21: xuan ji
CV 22: XIII 22: tian tu
CV 23: XIII 23: lian quan
CV 24: XIII 24: cheng jiang
GB 2 (GB 2): VII 2: ting hui
GB 12: VII 12: wan gu
GB 14: VII 14: yang bai
GB 20: VII 20: feng chi

GB 21: VII 21: jian jing
GB 23: VII 23: zhe jin
GB 24: VII 24: ri yue
GB 25: VII 25: jing men
GB 26: VII 26: dai mai
GB 30: VII 30: huan tiao
GB 31: VII 31: feng shi
GB 34: VII 34: yang ling guan
GB 35: VII 35: yang jiao
GB 37: VII 37: guang ming
GB 38: VII 38: yang fu
GB 39: VII 39: xuan zhong
GB 40: VII 40: qiu xu
GB 41: VII 41: zu lin ch'i
GB 42: VII 42: di wu hui
GB 43: VII 43: jia xi
GB 44: VII 44: zu qiao yin
GV 1 (GV 1): XIV 1: chang qiang
GV 2 (GV 2): XIV 2: yao shu
GV 3 (GV 3): XIV 3: yao yang
  guan
GV 4 (GV 4): XIV 4: ming men
GV 6 (GV 6): XIV 6: ji zhong
GV 9 (GV 9): XIV 9: zhi yang
GV 10: XIV 10: ling tai
GV 12: XIV 12: shen zhu
GV 13: XIV 13: tao dao
GV 14: XIV 14: da zhui
GV 15: XIV 15: ya men
GV 16: XIV 16: feng fu
GV 17: XIV 17: nao hu
GV 20: XIV 20: bai hui
GV 23: XIV 23: shang xing
GV 26: XIV 26: ren zhong
Ht 1: I 1: ji quan
Ht 2: I 2: qing ling
Ht 3: I 3: xiao hai
Ht 4: I 4: ling dao
Ht 5: I 5: tong li
Ht 6: I 6: yin xi
Ht 7: I 7: shen men
Ht 8: I 8: xiao fu

Ht 9: I 9: xiao chong

K 1 (K 1): IV 1: yong guan

K 2 (K 2): IV 2: ran gu

K 3 (K 3): IV 3: tai xi

K 4 (K 4): IV 4: da zhong

K 5 (K 5): IV 5: shui quan

K 6 (K 6): IV 6: zhao hai

K 7 (K 7): IV 7: fu liu

K 8 (K 8): IV 8: jiao xin

K 9 (K 9): IV 9: zhu bin

K 10: IV 10: yin gu

K 12: IV 12: da he

K 13: IV 13: ch'i xue

K 14: IV 14: si man

K 16: IV 16: huang shu

K 19: IV 19: yin du

K 24: IV 24: ling xu

K 25: IV 25: shen cang

K 27: IV 27: shu fu

LI 1 (LI 1): X 1: shang yang

LI 2 (LI 2): X 2: er jian

LI 3 (LI 3): X 3: san jian

LI 4 (LI 4): X 4: he gu

LI 5 (LI 5): X 5: yang xi

LI 6 (LI 6): X 6: pian li

LI 7 (LI 7): X 7: wen liu

LI 10: X 10: shou san li

LI 11: X 11: qu chi

LI 14: X 14: bi nao

LI 15: X 15: jian yu

LI 16: X 16: ju gu

LI 18: X 18: fu tu

LI 19: X 19: he liao

LI 20: X 20: ying xiang

Lu 1 (Lu 1): IX 1: zhong fu

Lu 2 (Lu 2): IX 2: yun men

Lu 3 (Lu 3): IX 3: tian fu

Lu 5 (Lu 5): IX 5: chi ze

Lu 6 (Lu 6): IX 6: kong zui

Lu 7 (Lu 7): IX 7: lie que

Lu 8 (Lu 8): IX 8: jing qu

Lu 9 (Lu 9): IX 9: tai yuan

Lu 10: IX 10: yu ji

Lu 11: IX 11: xiao shang

Lv 1 (Lv 1): VIII 1: da dun

Lv 2 (Lv 2): VIII 2: xing jian

Lv 3 (Lv 3): VIII 3: tai chong

Lv 4 (Lv 4): VIII 4: zhong feng

Lv 5 (Lv 5): VIII : li gou

Lv 6 (Lv 6): VIII 6: zhong du

Lv 7 (Lv 7): VIII 7: xi guan

Lv 8 (Lv 8): VIII 8: qu quan

Lv 13: VIII 13: zhang men

Lv 14: VIII 14: ch'i men

PC 1: V 1: tian chi

PC 2: V 2: tian guan

PC 3: V 3: qu ze

PC 4: V 4: xi men

PC 5: V 5: jian shi

PC 6: V 6: nei guan

PC 7: V 7: da ling

PC 8: V 8: lao gong

PC 9: V 9: zhong chong

SI 1 (SI 1): II 1: xiao ze

SI 2 (SI 2): II 2: qian gu

SI 3 (SI 3): II 3: hou xi

SI 4 (SI 4): II 4: wan gu

SI 5 (SI 5): II 5: yang gu

SI 6 (SI 6): II 6: yang lao

SI 7 (SI 7): II 7: zhi zheng

SI 8 (SI 8): II 8: xiao hai

SI 11: II 11: tian zong

SI 16: II 16: tian chuang

SI 19: II 19: ting gong

Sp 1 (Sp 1): XII 1: yin bai

Sp 2 (Sp 2): XII 2: da du

Sp 3 (Sp 3): XII 3: tai bei

Sp 4 (Sp 4): XII 4: gong sun

Sp 5 (Sp 5): XII 5: shang qiu

Sp 6 (Sp 6): XII 6: san yin jiao

Sp 8 (Sp 8): XII 8: di ji

Sp 9 (Sp 9): XII 9: yin ling quan

Sp 10: XII 10: xue hai

Sp 12: XI 12: que pen

Sp 12: XII 12: chong men
Sp 13: XII 13: fu she
Sp 15: XII 15: da heng
Sp 21: XII 21: da bao
St 2 (St 2): XI 2: si bai
St 4 (St 4): XI 4: di cang
St 6 (St 6): XI 6: jia che
St 7 (St 7): XI 7: xia guan
St 8 (St 8): XI 8: tou wei
St 9 (St 9): XI 9: ren ying
St 13: XI 13: ch'i hu
St 15: XI 15: wu yi
St 18: XI 18: ru gen
St 21: XI 21: liang men
St 23: XI 23: tai yi
St 25: XI 25: tian shu
St 28: XI 28: shui dao
St 29: XI 29: gui lai
St 30: XI 30: ch'i chong
St 34: XI 34: liang qiu
St 35: XI 35: du bi
St 36: XI 36: zu san li
St 37: XI 37: shang ju xu
St 38: XI 38: tiao kou
St 39: XI 39: xia ju xu
St 40: XI 40: feng long
St 41: XI 41: jie xi
St 42: XI 42: chong yang

St 43: XI 43: xian gu
St 44: XI 44: nei ting
St 45: XI 45: li dui
TW 1 (TW 1): VI 1: guan chong
TW 2 (TW 2): VI 2: ye men
TW 3 (TW 3): VI 3: zhong zhu
TW 4 (TW 4): VI 4: yang chi
TW 5 (TW 5): VI 5: wai guan
TW 6 (TW 6): VI 6: zhi gou
TW 7 (TW 7): VI 7: hui zong
TW 10: VI 10: tian jing
TW 14: VI 14: jian liao
TW 17: VI 17: yi feng
TW 21: VI 21: er men
TW 23: VI 23: si zhu kong
Luo xue: Luo Connecting points
Yuan xue: Source points
Chong Mai (Penetrating Vessel)
Dai Mai (Girdle Vessel)
Du Mai (Governing Vessel)
Ren Mai (Conception Vessel)
Yang Qiao Mai (Yang Motility
  Vessel)
Yang Wei Mai (Yang Linking
  Vessel)
Yin Qiao Mai (Yin Motility
  Vessel)
Yin Wei Mai (Yin Linking Vessel)

USEFUL ADDRESSES

USA

American Association of
    Acupuncture & Oriental
    Medicine
c/o National Acupuncture
    Headquarters
1424 16th Street, NW,
Suite 501
Washington DC 20036
Tel: (202) 332 5794

National Commission for the
    Certification of Acupuncturists
C/o 1424 16th Street, NW,
Suite 501
Washington DC 20036
Tel: (202) 332 5794

American Herbal Association
PO Box 1673
Nevada City
CA 95959

Australia

Australian College of Alternative
    Medicine
11 Howard Avenue
Mount Waverley
VIC 3149
Tel: (03) 807 4536

Australian College of Oriental
    Medicine
24 Price Road
Lalorma
VIC 3766
Tel: (03) 728 4073

Australian Traditional Medicine
  Society
120 Blaxland Road
Ryde
NSW 2112
Tel: (02) 809 6800

Australian Acupuncture
  Association Ltd
PO Box 5142
West End, Brisbane, Australia,
  4101
Tel: +61 7 3846 5866 (outside
  Australia)
freecall 1800 025 334 (within
  Australia)
Fax: (07) 3846 5276
Email: aaca@eis.net.au

Queensland Institute of Natural
  Science
PO Box 82
Mapleton
QLD 4560
Tel: (074) 429 377

New Zealand

Holistic Health Centre
CPO Box 2273
Auckland
Tel: (09) 307 2588

Canada

Acupuncture Foundation of
  Canada Institute
AFCI, 2131 Lawrence Avenue
  East, Ste. 204
Scarborough, ON M1R 5G4
Canada
Tel: 416-752-3988
Fax: 416-752-4398
Email: info@afcinstitute.com

Singapore

Singapore Thong Chai Medical
  Institute
Thong Chai Building
50 Chin Swee Road
01-0 Singapore 0316
02-0 Tel: (65) 733 6905

United Kingdom

Council for Acupuncture
179 Gloucester Place
London NW1 6DX
Tel: 0171 724 5330

Registry of Chinese Medicine
19 Trinity Road
London N2 8JJ
Tel: 0181 883 8432

The British Acupuncture Council
Park House
206-208 Latimer Road
London W10 6RE
Tel: 0181 964 0222
Fax: 0181 964 0333

Healthworks Ltd.
30-38 Dock Street
Leeds
Tel: +44 (0)113 2346624
Fax: +44 (0)113 242 7782
Email: info@d-access.demon.co.uk
internet: http://www.health-
works.co.uk

You can also obtain a considerable amount of information from the
World Wide Web. Listed below are some typical 'net' addresses that
may prove useful.

Research into the Practice of Traditional Chinese Medicine in
Victoria
Tender Brief No. 335 Research into the Practice of Traditional
Chinese Medicine in Victoria. Contents: 1. Background 2. National
Directions 3. Victorian Review of Traditional Chinese ...
http://hna.ffh.vic.gov.au/phb/hce/chinese.html

Press Release for Traditional Chinese Medicine & Pharmacology
Traditional Chinese Medicine & Pharmacology Press Release 10,000
years in the Making Hopkins Technology's new CD-ROM, Traditional
Chinese Medicine & Pharmacology, took over 10,000 ...
http://www.hoptechno.com/cherblpr.htm

China Institute of Traditional Chinese Medicine
China Institute of Traditional Chinese Medicine specialises in traditional Chinese medicine
http://www.pageindex.com/c/china.htm

Traditional Chinese Medicine and Cancer
How is cancer regarded in traditional Chinese medicine? What causes the cancer according to TCM? How does herbal medicine treat cancer? How can you get further help? Return to Info ...
http://www.generation.net/~cathay/xcancer.html

Centennial College offers training in traditional chinese medicine
Canada News Wire Give us your message. We'll give you the world. Attention Health/Lifestyle Editors: Centennial College offers training in traditional Chinese medicine, Scarborough
http://www.newswire.ca/releases/January1996/22/c2353.html

Traditional Chinese Medicine Programs
Traditional Chinese Medicine Multimedia Program CD Chinese Acupuncture and Moxibustion Compilation of Channels and Acupoints Chinese Herbs Chinese Healthcare Massage Traditional ...
http://www.china-guide.com/ad-medic.htm

Studies On Alternative Medicine Traditional Chinese Medicine. 1 UI - 96057897 AU – Hijikata Y AU – Kaneko J AU - Xi L AU – Nasu M AU – Yamashita S IN – Tokyo Adventist Hospital, Japan. TI – Traditional Chinese medicines improve the course of ...
http://www.libraries.wayne.edu/shiffman/altmed/therapy/stu_chi.html

Alpine Health – Traditional Chinese Medicine Homepage
Traditional Chinese Medicine What Is It? The Five Elements Vital Substances Herbal Supplements And How They Work Home / The Story / Traditional Chinese Medicine / Products / Wholesale ...
http://www.alpinehealth.com/mk.html

Home Page of ACTCM
Home Page of ACTCM Health Care for the Next Century American College of Traditional Chinese Medicine American College of Traditional Chinese Medicine(ACTCM) : 455 Arkansas Street San
http://www.iijnet.or.jp/GOTO/engdocs/actcm.

The Program Master's Degree in Traditional Chinese Medicine Five Branches
Institute is dedicated to the transmission of traditional Chinese medicine to the West. Our program is designed to train practitioners who will represent a new synthesis of both ...
http://www.w3wiz.com/fivebranches/curr.html

Media Mart CD-ROM *Traditional Chinese Medicine* (PC/MAC)
Hopkins Technology
Media Mart Selection *Traditional Chinese Medicine* (PC/MAC) CDX #105672 Hopkins Technology $32.99 Comprehensive text on Chinese traditional medicine. Comparisons of modern Western ...
http://www.netvideo.com/mediamart/cdrom/ref/sku/mm105672.html

Traditional Chinese Medicine
is preventative medicine based on the yin-yang principle. Everyone is a combination of yin and yang. Your goal is to maintain a balance of yin and yang (through proper diet, exercise, ...
http://www.moysginseng.com/medicine.html

Traditional Chinese Medicine and Pharmacology
Comprehensive text on Chinese traditional medicine. Comparisons of modern Western medicine and science to traditional Chinese medicine. Text and diagrams such as yin and yang and the ...
http://turboguide.com/cdprod1/cdhrec/008/978.shtml

Book Store
TCM Products Traditional Chinese Medicine Chinese Economy Chinese Culture Journals and Papers TCM Products. Series Models of Chinese Acupuncture Points CD-ROM: Traditional ...
http://www.china-invest.com/books.html

Traditional Chinese Medicine
This article submitted by Julie Leibel on 9/14/96. Author's Email: jleibel@cyberatl.net I had wonderful success in treatment for Shingles, and other problems with traditional Chinese ...
http://neuro-
www.mgh.harvard.edu/neurowebforum/GeneralFeedbackArticles/Tra
ditionalChineseMedicine.htm

Health: *Basic Knowledge of Traditional Chinese Medicine*, Zhang Dazhao and Wu Xiaolong. A clear and easy to understand introduction to the basic principles and theories of traditional
http://www.chinabooks.com/Catalog/health.html

Traditional Chinese Medicine
Comprehensive text on Chinese traditional medicine. Comparisons of modern Western medicine and science to traditional Chinese medicine. Text and diagrams such as yin and yang http://turboguide.com/cdprod1/cdhrec/010/982.shtml

Chinese Medicine Under the Microscope – Tehan
The State Government and practitioners of traditional Chinese medicine have joined forces to launch a comprehensive study of its application in Victoria. The Health Minister, Mrs ...
http://www.dpc.vic.gov.au/pressrel/4436.htm

A brief introduction to Fujian University of Traditional Chinese Medicine
You can also see the message in Chinese GB code or BIG-5 code. Founded in 1958, Fujian University of Traditional Chinese Medicine is located in the hot spring area in Fuzhou. In the ...
http://china-window.com/Fujian_w/edu/tcm/etcm.html

Traditional Chinese Medical Journals and Periodicals
Alternative Medicine Journal. Prime National Publishing Corp. 470 Boston Post Road, Weston, MA 02193 U.S.A. 617/899-2702 Alternative Therapies in Health and Medicine. Inno Vision PO ...
http://www.acupuncture.com/TCMSchools/Sub.htm

Traditional Chinese Medicine
(TCM) is at least 6,000 years old. Objects dated from 4,000 BC are considered the earliest needles used in acupuncture. While they were only stones, bones, wood and bamboo, they ...
http://graddiv.ucsb.edu/~nivens/herbs/tcm.html

Examples from Traditional Chinese Medicine and Pharmacology CD-ROM
Ephedra (Mahuang) Pharmaceutical Name: Herba Ephedrae Botanical Name: 1. Ephedra sinica Stapf; 2. Ephedra equisetina Bunge; 3. Ephedra intermedia Schrenk et Mey. Common Name: Ephedra, ...
http://webster.skypoint.net/members/pdunn/cherbex1.htm

Institute for Traditional Medicine – Traditional Chinese Medicine
ITM Online Resources for the Study of Chinese Medicine [IMAGE] Information Available Here: Resources for the study of Chinese Medicine: Schools & Institutes Resources for the study of
http://www.europa.com/~itm/resource.htm

The Acupuncture Foundation of Canada Institute
Contact:
Cheryl A. Kwok, Executive Director
AFCI, 2131 Lawrence Avenue East, Ste. 204
Scarborough, ON M1R 5G4 Canada
Tel: 416-752-3988. Fax: 416-752-4398. Email: info@afcinstitute.com

The British Acupuncture Council
Park House
206-208 Latimer Road
London W10 6RE
Tel: 0181 964 0222
Fax: 0181 964 0333

The Medical Acupuncture Web Page
The Medical Acupuncture Web Page runs on the WWW server of the
medical school at Aristotle University of Thessaloniki.
Email : karanik@med.auth.gr

Australian Acupuncture Association Ltd
Contact Details
Post: PO Box 5142
West End, Brisbane, Australia, 4101
Tele: +61 7 3846 5866 (outside Australia)
Freecall 1800 025 334 (within Australia)
Fax: (07) 3846 5276
Email: aaca@eis.net.au

The Acupuncture Home Page can be found at:
http: //www.rscom.com/tcm/

Foundation for Traditional Chinese Medicine
122a Acomb Road
York YO2 4EY
Tel: (01904) 785120 / 784828

FURTHER READING

Acupuncture, Peter Mole, Element Books, 1992

Acupuncture, Meridian Theory and Acupuncture Points, by Li Ding, Pacific View Press, 1992

Alternative Medicine, Dr Andrew Stanway, Bloomsbury Books, 1979

Altas of Therapeutic Motion for Treatment and Health: A Guide to traditional Chinese massage and exercise therapy, Ed. Sun Shuchun, Foreign Language Press, 1989

Between Heaven and Earth, Harriet and Efrem Korngold-Beinfield, Ballantine, 1991

Charts of Meridians and their Points, by Li Ding, Foreign Language Press, 1990

Chinese Acupuncture and Moxibustion, Dr Cui Yongqiang and Dr Chen Ken, Foreign Language Press, 1993

Chinese Acupuncture and Moxibustion, ed. Cheng Xinnong, Foreign Language Press, 1993

Chinese Bodywork: A complete manual of Chinese therapeutic massage, ed. Sun Chengnan, Pacific View Press, 1993

Chinese Family Acupoint Massage, by Wang Chuangui, Foreign Language Press, 1992

Chinese Herbal Medicine, Richard Craze & Stephen Tang, Piatkus, 1995

Chinese Herbal Prescriptions, Martin Palmer & Stephen Tang, Rider, 1986

Chinese Massage Therapy, ed. Sun Chengnan, Shandong Science and Tech. Press, 1992

Chinese Medicine: The web that has no weaver, Ted Kaptchuk, Congdon and Weed/Rider, 1983

Chinese Tui Na Therapy, Wang Fu, Foreign Language Press, 1994

Clinical Handbook of Chinese Prepared Medicines, Chun Lan Zhu, Paradigm Publications, 1989

The Complete New Herbal, Richard Mabey, Elm Tree Books, 1988

The Essential Book of Traditional Chinese Medicine, Liu Yan Chi, Columbia University Press, 1988

Essentials of Chinese Diagnostics, Manfred Porkert, Chinese Medical Publications, 1983

Feng Shui for Beginners, Richard Craze, Hodder & Stoughton, 1994

Fighting Drug Abuse with Acupuncture: The treatment that works, Ellinor R. Mitchell, Pacific View Press, 1996

Finger Acupressure, by Doctor P. C. Chan, Life & Health Books, 1990

Five Elements and Ten Stems, Kikko Matsumoto, Paradigm Publications, 1983

Fundamentals of Chinese Acupuncture, Andrew Ellis, Paradigm Publications, 1989

Healing Plants, Manfried Pahlow, Barron's Educational Series, 1993

How to Treat Yourself with Chinese Herbs, Dr Hong Yen Hsu, Keats Publishing, 1993

In the Footsteps of the Yellow Emperor: Tracing the History of Traditional Acupuncture, Peter Eckman, M.D., Ph.D., M.Ac., Cypress 1996

The Miracle of Acupuncture, Xu Xi, Foreign Language Press, 1993

The Practical Application of Meridian Style Acupuncture, John E. Pirog, Pacific View Press, 1994

Selecting the Right Acupoints: A handbook on acupuncture therapy, Geng Junying, New World Press,1995

The Yellow Emperor's Classic of Internal Medicine, ed. Ilza Veith, University of California Press, 1972

Zang Fu, Jeremy Ross, Churchill Livingstone, 1983

Zhu's Scalp Acupuncture, Mingqing Zhu, trans. Dale Chow, Yuansheng Zhang, Eight Dragon Publications, 1992

INDEX